RENAL DIET COOKBOOK FOR BEGINNERS 2021:

How to Avoid Life-Threatening Consequences and Protect Your Kidneys from Dialysis. Manage Your Lifestyle Effectively While Enjoying Your Favorite Recipes

© Copyright 2020 - All rights reserved.

Table of Contents

Introduction

R enal failure is more often than not, difficult to predict or even prevent. But you can certainly lower your risk of renal failure by taking good care of your kidneys. To take proper care of your kidneys, here are the things you should keep in mind:

Whenever you are buying any over the counter medication, you should pay close attention to the labels. You should always follow instructions given on these over-the-counter medicines like aspirin, ibuprofen and acetaminophen. Taking an excess of pain medications would increase the risk of renal failure, and this is more likely when you already have a pre-existing kidney disease, or some other problem like diabetes or high blood pressure.

You should work hand-in-hand with your doctor for managing your kidney problems. If you have a pre-existing condition, or any other disease, the risk of kidney failure increases; especially when you have diabetes, high blood pressure or any other kidney related problem. Therefore, you should stay on track with your treatment and follow the doctor's recommendations for managing your condition. You should make living healthy your lifestyle choice and priority. Keep yourself active, stay fit by exercising regularly, eat a balanced diet, and consume alcohol in moderation (if you drink).

There is so much you can do to keep your kidneys healthy and have them functioning properly. Here are some more tips you should keep in mind to ensure proper functioning of your kidneys:

Make sure that you are always sufficiently hydrated, but do not overdo this. There are no studies that conclude that over-hydration is good for enhancing the performance of your kidneys. It is definitely good to drink sufficient water, and you can drink around four to six glasses of water per day. Consuming more water than this will definitely not help your kidneys perform better. In fact, it would just increase the stress on your kidneys!

Your kidneys are capable of tolerating a wide variety of dietary habits, and usually most of the kidney problems crop up from other existing medical conditions like high blood pressure or diabetes. Because of this, it would be advisable for you to eat foods that will help you regulate your weight and blood pressure. If you were able to prevent diabetes and even high blood pressure, then your kidneys would be healthy as well.

If you are already consuming foods that are healthy, then it would also make sense for you to exercise regularly. This is because regular physical activity will prevent weight gain and also regulate your blood pressure. But you should be careful about how much exercise you do, especially if you aren't used to exercising. Don't overexert yourself if you are just getting started, because this would just increase the pressure on your kidneys and could lead to the breaking down of your muscles.

CHAPTER 1:

What Is A Renal Diet?

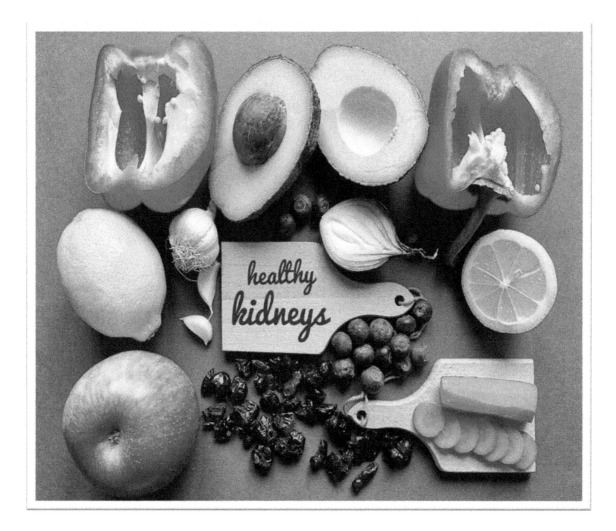

The renal diet is a type of diet designed to bring relief to patients with damaged or slow renal functions and chronic kidney diseases. There is no a single uniformed type of renal diet—this is the case because the requirements of renal diet, as well as the restrictions need to match the needs of the patient, and be based on what the doctors have prescribed for the patient's overall health.

However, all forms of renal diet have one thing in common: they improve your renal functions, bring some relief to your kidneys, and prevent kidney disease in patients with numerous risk factors. All this put together improves your overall health and well-being. The grocery list we have provided will help you know the groceries you should introduce to your diet, and which groups of food should be avoided in order to improve your kidney's performance. That way, you can start shopping for your new lifestyle.

You don't need to shop for many different types of groceries all at once, as it is always better to use fresh produce; although frozen food also makes a good alternative when fresh fruit and vegetables are not available.

Remember to treat canned goods as suggested; it is recommended you drain excess liquid from the canned food.

As far as the renal diet we are recommending in our guide, this form of kidney-friendly dietary regimen offers a solution in form of low-sodium and low-potassium meals and groceries. This is why we are also offering simple and easy renal diet recipes in our guide. Do follow the dietary plan compiled for all stages of renal system failure, unless your doctor expressly forbids you from taking some of the groceries we have listed in our ultimate grocery list for renal patients.

CHAPTER 2:

Importance of Sodium, Potassium, Phosphorous and Low Salt

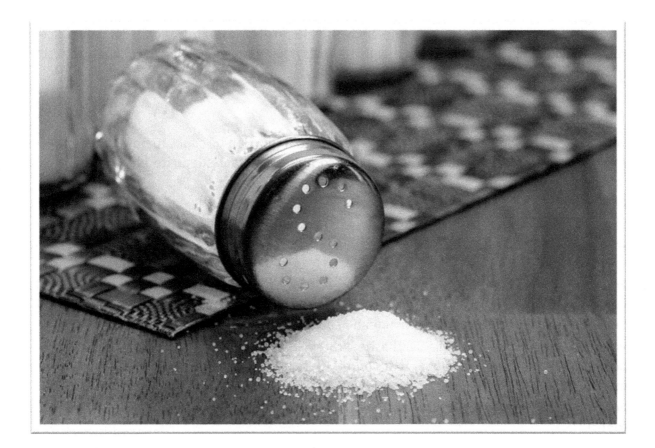

The Role of Sodium in the Body

Sodium is one of the elements necessary for the proper functioning of the body. It is primarily responsible for water and electrolyte management, but also has other functions. What are these other roles?

Are there serious effects of sodium excess or deficiency?

How do we introduce a diet that will allow us reduce sodium intake?

Sodium has important functions in the body, and disturbances in its concentration can cause serious problems. The main tasks of this valuable element include:

- Maintaining the osmotic balance in the extracellular fluids of the body - this means that it regulates the volume of water in the body and protects us from dehydration.

- Maintaining acid-base balance (this it does together with potassium and chlorine).
- Involved in the conduction of nerve impulses - sodium is a potassium antagonist, and this element creates a concentration difference on both sides of the cell membrane. This enables the transmission of impulses. This process is responsible for the state of smooth muscle, skeletal and heart tension.
- Participation in the process of glucose and amino acid transport across cell membranes.
- Activating salivary amylase (a digestive enzyme present in saliva).

Normal sodium concentration in the body is 135 to 145 mmol/l, and its maintenance is responsible for the renin-angiotensin-aldosterone system (a complex hormonal enzyme system that also regulates the volume of water in the body).

The Role of Potassium in the Body

Potassium is an element that performs many essential functions. Thanks to potassium, our cells can transmit electrical impulses. Potassium also helps maintain adequate blood pressure and muscle tone.

Potassium, as an electrolyte, also controls muscle function. It enables the generation of electrical impulses in the cells of our body, and even in the cells of heart muscles. In other words, it is responsible for each heartbeat. Potassium also plays the same function in skeletal muscles.

Potassium is a sodium antagonist, and its opposite action reduces the volume of extracellular fluids, which helps to control the amount of water in the body. This role of potassium has also been associated with the ability to maintain healthy blood pressure by lowering it.

Potassium also helps our cells synthesize proteins, which are muscle building blocks. Thus, potassium is one of the elements that control muscle building and help us maintain a healthy muscle mass.

Potassium, being also a calcium antagonist, is responsible for proper muscle tone (so-called tonus).

Also, potassium helps maintain acid-base balance, thus maintaining the homeostasis of the whole body.

Potassium and Our Health

For our body to function properly, balance must be maintained between potassium and sodium. Disorders in the concentrations of these macroelements cause the occurrence of one of the most common and severe diseases known to man - hypertension and heart disease. Unlike sodium, low potassium levels promote these diseases.

It is rare that people suffer from potassium deficiency or bearing. This happens, however, in cases where the functioning of our body is disturbed.

Potassium deficiency, or hypokalemia, can occur when we use high blood pressure diuretics. It also occurs when there is prolonged vomiting or diarrhea, and can also be caused by some kidney problems. Symptoms of hypokalemia are weak, flaccid muscles, arrhythmias, and a slight increase in blood pressure.

Hyperkalemia, which is a higher than normal level of potassium, can cause a dangerous arrhythmia. Hyperkalemia occurs when the kidneys are weak, infections are severe, or when you are taking some heart medicines.

The Role of Phosphorus in the Body

Because as much as 85% of phosphorus is found in bones and teeth, it is necessary to maintain their proper structure. It also occurs in soft tissues and cell membranes, like the tissues of the muscles, heart and brain. It also plays an essential role in the process of growth and reconstruction or repair of damaged tissues. As one of the elements that take part in the processes occurring in the human body, phosphorus is also an energy transmitter. Thanks to this mineral, food is converted into energy that translates into muscle work.

Phosphorus also ensures the proper functioning of nerves and the brain. It is involved in many chemical reactions and metabolic processes in our body. It also maintains the overall vitality of the body. In addition, it plays an important role in the work of the heart. For researchers, it is an important carrier of genetic information because it is a component of DNA.

CHAPTER 3:

Kidney Disease And How To Avoid Dialysis

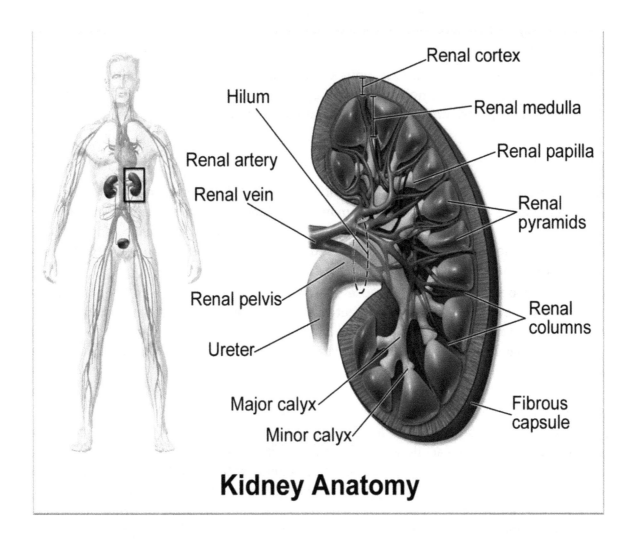

Kidney Anatomy

When you educate yourself about chronic kidney disease, you will feel more empowered and less scared about living with the disease. You can take back control of your life! What you eat and the lifestyle choices you make are very important. If you are diagnosed in the early stages of the disease, there are many steps you can take to prolong your kidney function. When you make positive changes, have patience, and commit to working closely with your healthcare team, there is a good chance that you will be able to enjoy a high-quality, happy and active life.

What Is Kidney Disease?

Let's begin by understanding how kidneys function. Your body has two kidneys that are bean-shaped and about the size of your fist. When the kidneys are working properly, they help keep your whole body in balance by performing the following important tasks:

1. Clean waste materials from your blood.
2. Remove excess water from your body.
3. Regulate your blood pressure.
4. Stimulate your bone marrow to make red blood cells.
5. Control the amount of calcium and phosphorus absorbed and excreted.

When you have chronic kidney disease, your kidneys do not work properly and cannot perform these tasks. Although there is no cure for kidney failure, it is very possible to live a long and healthy life with proper treatment and good dietary and lifestyle choices.

Causes

Kidney disease is most often caused by poorly controlled diabetes or high blood pressure. Physical injury and drug toxicity can also damage your kidneys. Kidney disease affects people of all ages and races; but Hispanics, African Americans, and Native Americans tend to have a greater risk of kidney failure. This is mostly due to a higher incidence of diabetes and high blood pressure in these populations.

Uncontrolled diabetes is the primary cause of kidney failure. In fact, 44% of people who start dialysis have kidney failure because of diabetes. Diabetes develops when blood glucose (blood sugar) levels are too high in the body. When our bodies digest protein from the food we eat, the process of digestion creates waste products. In the kidneys, millions of small blood vessels, called capillaries, act as filters. As blood flows through the capillaries, the waste products are filtered out into our urine. Substances such as protein and red blood cells are too big to pass through the capillaries and stay in the blood.

Diabetes damages this process. Too much blood is filtered when there is a high levels of blood sugar. All the extra work wears down the filters, and after many years, the filters start to leak. The good protein our bodies need is then filtered out and lost through the urine. Eventually, the kidneys cannot remove the extra waste from the blood. This ultimately leads to kidney damage or failure. This damage can happen over many years without any signs or symptoms. That is why it is so important for people with diabetes to manage their blood-sugar levels and get tested for kidney disease periodically.

High blood pressure is another contributor to kidney disease. One in three Americans with high blood pressure, also known as hypertension, is at risk for kidney disease. High blood pressure is the second leading cause of kidney disease and increases your risk of developing a heart attack or stroke. Treatment and lifestyle changes, including blood-pressure medications, following a healthy diet, and exercising can lower blood pressure.

High blood pressure means the heart has to work harder at pumping blood. As time passes, high blood pressure can harm blood vessels in your body, including the ones in your kidneys—which causes them to stop filtering out waste and extra fluid from your body. The extra fluid in your blood vessels can also make your blood pressure rise, creating a vicious and detrimental cycle. As in diabetes, this damage can happen over many years without any signs or symptoms. It is very important for people with high blood pressure to control their blood pressure and get tested for kidney disease, just like people who have diabetes. High blood pressure is the cause of more than 25,000 new cases of kidney failure in the United States every year.

Symptoms

Kidney failure is a progressive disease; it does not happen overnight. Some people in the early stages of kidney disease do not show any symptoms. Symptoms usually appear in the upcoming stages of kidney disease. Some people may not even show any symptoms of kidney disease until their kidneys fail (end stage).

When the kidneys are damaged, wastes and toxins can build up in your body. Once the buildup starts to occur, you may feel sick and experience some of the following symptoms:

- Nausea
- Weakness
- Poor appetite
- Trouble sleeping
- Itching
- Tiredness
- Weight loss
- Swelling of your feet and ankles
- Muscle cramps (especially in the legs)
- Anemia (low red blood cell count)

The good news is that once you begin treatment for kidney disease, your symptoms and general health will start to improve!

Stages of Chronic Kidney Disease (CKD)

There are five stages of CKD. Each level has a corresponding GFR index that accompanies it. It is very important for someone who has CKD to have continual monitoring of their GFR index because it doesn't take much for the change in the index to trigger the following stage of chronic kidney disease. For this reason alone, it is important to monitor what you are eating in conjunction with your stage of disease.

Stage 1 and 2 CKD (Normal to High and Mild GFR)

Most people who have stage one or two chronic kidney disease do not know that they have it. Their GFR index is generally greater than ninety milliliters per minute for stage one, and an index that is sixty to eighty-nine milliliters per minute for stage two. Generally, the people who have been diagnosed with stage one or two CKD were diagnosed because of tests for another illness.

Symptoms of stage one and two can be extremely vague, but a good indicator is higher than normal creatinine levels in the blood or urine. With stage two, the filtration levels of the kidney have begun to decrease, but not at an overly noticeable level. People living with stage one and two CKD can still live a normal life, they can't cure their kidneys, but they can help stop or slow the progression of the disease. Keeping blood pressure in line and eating a diet that is renal friendly are good first steps. Your doctor will keep up on your creatine levels and GFR to monitor the progression of CKD.

Stage 3A and 3B (Moderate GFR)

Stage three is broken up into two GFR indexes, but the symptoms aren't much different. The GFR index for stage A is an index of forty-five to fifty-nine milliliters per minute. The GFR for stage B is thirty to forty-four milliliters per minute. As the kidney's functions decrease, the build-up of wastes causes the body to go into uremia, which is a buildup of that waste in the blood. More complications from kidney failure become apparent. The chances for high blood pressure increase, and patients are likely to exhibit anemia. Swelling, or edema, may start to become apparent because of the water retention and typically starts in the arms and legs. Diet becomes increasingly more important with stage three CDK due to the buildup in the body.

Stage 4 (Severe GFR)

Stage four is the last stop before kidney failure. The GFR index for stage four is fifteen to twenty-nine milliliters per minute. Stage four patients are more than likely receiving dialysis and are thinking about transplant in the near future. The body is barely filtering the wastes, hence the need for mechanical intervention for filtration. At this stage, edema worsens, and physical symptoms can be overwhelming. Diet in this phase is stricter and will consist of limiting things that can build up in the body which the kidneys are no longer able to take care of on their own.

Stage 5 (End Stage GFR)

Once the kidneys are no longer filtering the waste in the body, dialysis will be necessary to live. The GFR index in end-stage is less than fifteen milliliters per minute. There is also a chance that if you meet qualifications, you will be put on a transplant list. Stage five CKD leaves the patient feeling sick almost all of the time because of the toxins and waste built up in the body. A nephrologist, a doctor who specializes in treating kidneys, will be a permanent part of your medical regimen. Diet will be an absolute must, as well as limiting fluid intake.

How To Naturally Prevent the need for Dialysis

Dialysis steps in as a last case scenario when both kidneys lose sufficient function to clean the blood. Before the toxicity reaches a damaging level, it must be eradicated through external sources. Individuals who suffer from acute kidney diseases end up going through dialysis to get their blood cleaned through the artificial dialysis machine. This dialysis machine mimics the role of our kidneys, and the blood is pumped into the machine, and then it is pumped back into the body simultaneously.

Those who never went through dialysis should know that it is one long and exhaustive process which every renal patient hates to go through. Fortunately, there are some effective measures to avoid dialysis. This precautionary measure can stop the progression of renal disease and even cure it to some extent.

- Exercise regularly
- Avoid excess salt in your diet
- Don't smoke
- Control of diabetes
- Control high blood pressure
- Eat correctly and lose excess weight
- Talk with your health care team

CHAPTER 4:

What Can You Eat And Drink

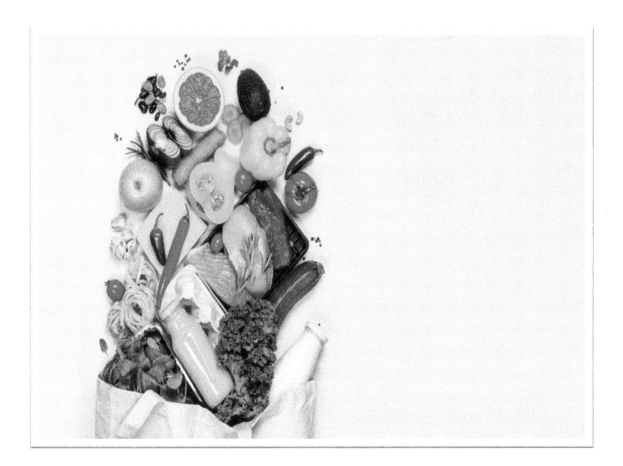

Low in Sodium

- Fresh and frozen portions of lamb, poultry, beef, fish, shrimp and pork.
- Fish and poultry; canned fish labeled as low sodium
- Eggs/egg substitutes
- Dried peas (not canned beans)
- Low sodium peanut butter, almond, rice, coconut milk and plant-based yogurts.
- Low sodium cream cheese and low sodium cheeses (like parmesan and ricotta).
- Ready-to-eat cereals
- Rolls and bread that are not salted.

- Almond, coconut, whole wheat, low sodium plain and all-purpose white flour; low sodium corn and tortillas.
- Low sodium breadsticks, crackers, unsalted popcorn and chips.
- Pasta and rice cooked without salt and low sodium noodles.
- Frozen or fresh vegetables; low sodium canned vegetables without seasoning or sauce.
- Low sodium vegetable juices, V-8 and low sodium tomato juice.
- Low sodium pickles
- Fresh potatoes or unsalted and unseasoned frozen french fries and mashed potatoes.
- Fresh and frozen canned fruits dried fruits.
- Low sodium salsa
- Low sodium soups that are canned.
- Homemade broths made without salt and fresh ingredients.
- Homemade pasta (without salt)
- Low sodium soy sauce
- Low sodium seasoning and marinades.
- Low sodium salad dressings
- Low sodium mayonnaise
- Unsalted butter, margarine and vegetable oils.
- Unsalted homemade ketchup.
- Unsalted mustard

Low in Potassium

- Asparagus, kale, broccoli, cucumber, zucchini, carrots, cabbage, bell pepper, eggplant, garlic and lettuce.
- Apples, grapes, pineapple, peaches, plum, all berries, watermelon.
- Rice milk
- Greens beans and snow peas
- White rice and bread that isn't whole.
- Dried cranberries
- Unsalted popcorn
- Hash browns and mashed potatoes made up of leached potatoes.
- Low sodium tomato and V-8 juice
- Unsalted sauces and apple sauce
- Unsalted noodles and pasta
- Non-dairy creams
- Sherbet
- Lemon and vanilla flavors (instead of chocolate)

Low in Phosphorus

- Celery, radishes, and baby carrots
- Apples, cherries, peaches, pineapples, blueberries and strawberries
- Pot roast beef, sirloin steak
- Skinless chicken and turkey (breast and thighs)
- Pork chop (mostly lean pork patty and pork roast)
- Veal chop
- Wild salmon, mahi-mahi, king crab, lobster, snow crab, oyster shrimp and water or oil-packed canned tuna.
- Plain bread (without salt), Italian bread, blueberry bread, sourdough bread, white bread, flatbread, wheat bread, pita bread, and cinnamon bread.
- Flour tortillas, corn tortillas.
- English muffins
- Macron, egg and rice noodles, spaghetti
- Couscous, long-grain white rice
- Cottage, blue, feta, parmesan and cream cheese
- Almond, soy and rice milk
- Non-dairy creamer
- Sorbet
- Pasteurized egg whites
- Unsalted popcorn

Kidney-Friendly Protein Options Which Are Included in the Overall Diet

- Lean beef and turkey
- Meat substitutes, like tofu and veggie sausage.
- Skinless chicken breast and thigh
- Salmon, trout, mackerel fish and shrimp
- Pork chops
- Cottage cheese
- Pasteurized eggs
- Greek yogurt
- Shakes made with rice, almond, coconut or soy milk.

Kidney-Friendly Fluid Options Which Are Included in This Diet

- Fruits like apples, cherries, grapes, berries, peaches and plums.
- Vegetables such as zucchini, cucumber, broccoli, cauliflower, cabbage, bell peppers, carrots, celery, lettuce and eggplant.
- Tea and coffee

- Gelatin
- Ice cubes
- Fruit juices
- Popsicles
- Milk substitutes
- Sherbet
- Low sodium soups

CHAPTER 5:

Forbidden Foods

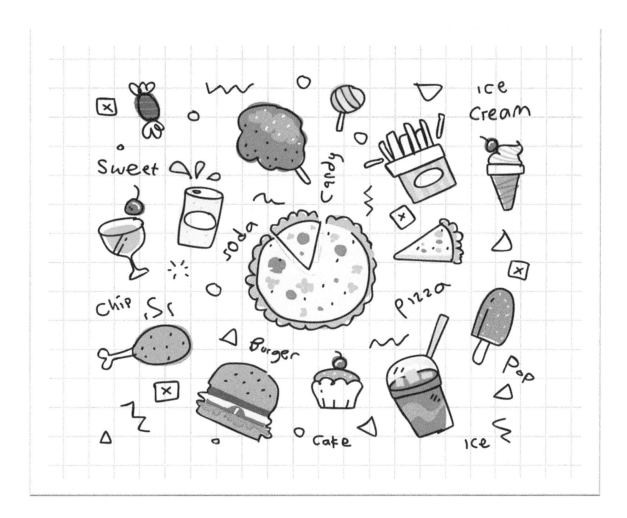

High in Sodium Foods That You Need to Avoid

- Different meats and sausages: chicken, pork, and cuts that have been preserved, smoked or cured.
- Fishes and seafood that are preserved
- Frozen dinners or packed dinners
- Canned food items like pasta or soup
- Salted nuts
- Salted and canned beans

- Buttermilk
- Cheese, cheese products, processed cottage cheese.
- Quick bread and bread with extra salt
- Salted rolls
- Biscuits and pancakes made by self-rising flour or their mixes.
- Salted crackers
- Dough of pasta, potatoes and rice that is processed and packaged.
- Vegetables and vegetable juices in cans.
- Salted regular pickles as well as olives and other pickled vegetables.
- Vegetables made with pork products.
- Dough of hash browns and scalloped potatoes, which are processed and packaged.
- Quick pasta meals
- Processed ketchup
- Processed and salted mustard
- Processed salsa
- Dehydrated or regular soups in cans
- Processed or regular broths
- Cup noodles, processed and salted ramen mixes
- Soy sauce
- Seasoning salts
- Marinades that are salted
- Salad dressings in bottles, processed or regular
- Salad dressings with bacon
- Salted butter and margarine
- Instant custard or pudding
- Ready-to-eat cakes

High in Potassium Foods That You Need to Avoid

- Cooked spinach, artichokes, okra, broccoli, beets, fried onions and sweet potato
- Bananas, avocados, honeydew, mango, orange, pomegranate, prune, pumpkin, coconut and cantaloupe
- Buttermilk and shakes
- Beans (either baked or refried)
- Legumes (like lentils)
- Nuts (like walnuts and raisins)
- Granola
- Whole grains and bran
- Fast foods (like french fries and other salty foods)

- Processed meats
- Vegetable juices
- Processed sauces (like tomato sauce)
- Fruit juices such as pomegranate juice, prune juice
- Creamed soups.
- Yogurt (frozen and regular)
- Ice creams
- Chocolate sweet dishes

High in Phosphorus Foods That You Need to Avoid

- Some Vegetables
- Some Fruits
- Parts of chicken and other poultry
- Ham and other pork products
- Hunted animals
- Some Seafood
- Plain Bread
- Tortillas
- Muffins
- Some pasta
- Some types of rice
- Certain cheeses
- Milk
- Yogurt
- Ice cream
- Eggs
- Snacks

CHAPTER 6:

What Are The Top Ways To Set Your Diet

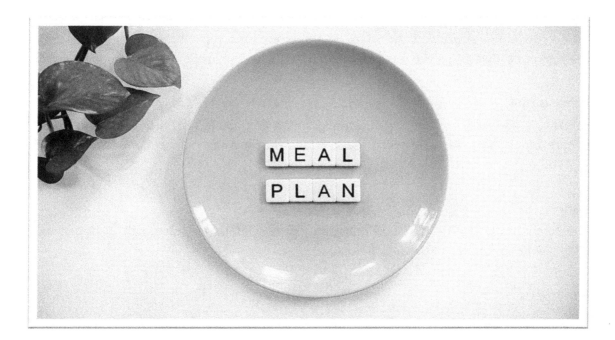

Meal Planning

Meal planning can make daily life easier all around but can be even more crucial to keeping up with a special diet. Make sure that when you are planning for meals, you leave a little bit of wiggle room for the unexpected schedule change. It is often better to use a small planner or datebook to write down the daily meals you plan on making. This can help you make your grocery list and can help you plan a budget. This can be a time-consuming project when you are first starting out; however, once you get into a routine of doing a meal plan, it can become quite easy. You can start by doing these:

- Make a list of kidney-friendly breakfasts, lunches and dinners. Consider what day of the week you will be planning for family dinners, what days you work, etc.
- Plan around current activities and plan only a week at a time, so you don't overwhelm yourself, and to help budget your meals more effectively.
- Watch sales ads. Most ads come out early enough in the week that you can plan for the following week and use them to their potential.
- Make effective lists. If you are having chicken for dinner on one night, but can get a better deal buying a larger quantity, precook the chicken and store it for another meal in the week.

Use your meal planner in conjunction with your food journal. This can help you use your eating habits to make healthier choices. If you prefer something sweet in the evening before bed, swap it out for fruit or something that is friendlier for your diet. If you find yourself snacking at your desk between meals, look into healthier alternatives like a hard candy that might occupy your oral fixation during that time.

Limiting Nutrient Intakes

A dietician or your doctor will be the one who sets limits for your diet and the amount you should be consuming every day. Included are the limits for a typical renal diet. These amounts may be higher or lower than the ones assigned to you, but they reflect the standard renal diet.

Phosphorus (mg)

Phosphorus is generally limited to 1000 milligrams a day. Generally, a doctor will prescribe a phosphate binder to take with your meals. Foods that are high in phosphorus include dark-colored sodas.

Potassium

Potassium should be limited to 2000 milligrams a day. Foods that are high in potassium are bananas, avocados, melons and black beans.

Sodium (mg)

Sodium intake amounts can vary, as a general rule of thumb, 2000 milligrams is typically the limit for renal diet patients. Sodium is something that is found in most foods and is a natural substance, so the best advice to take is "no added salt". Try using regular herbs in place of salting food. Salt substitutes also tend to be high in potassium, but if you are under on your potassium intake, they can be a nice alternative.

Protein (g)

Protein has an important role in the body. It fuels the body and helps it fight infections. Limiting protein consumption to only seven or eight ounces a day can help keep the body functioning but protect the kidneys from receiving too much.

Being Successful

Moderation is the key to any successful diet or lifestyle. Dietary guidelines promote eating all kinds of food, as long as they are enjoyed in moderation. This also holds true for a renal diet. You don't have to give up all the things that you love; you just have to monitor how much and how often you enjoy them. Keys to make the lifestyle change work are:

- Slow down while you are eating. It takes the body almost twenty minutes to send the signal to the brain that it is full. This is how people overeat, they eat too quickly, and the brain can't catch up until it is too late.

- Stop eating when you become full. It is okay to walk away from the table, feeling like you could eat more. Let your body tell you when it has had enough.
- Eat the cake but make it a small piece. Enjoy every bite, taste, and sensation of that piece of cake.
- If you are eating a large helping of something, especially in a restaurant, enjoy it. Eat half of it then and then take the rest home and enjoy it again the following day.
- You can reward yourself. Do it in moderation, though. Know what your body can and can't handle and use your food journal to alert you on where your levels stand for the day. It isn't just a tool, but more of an ally and best friend.

The goal of keeping track of everything is to turn the renal diet lifestyle into a marathon instead of a race. Keeping up with a lifestyle change that will be a permanent part of your life will be more encouraging than trying a short-term diet that can actually become psychologically harmful to your health.

CHAPTER 7:

Benefits of Renal Diet

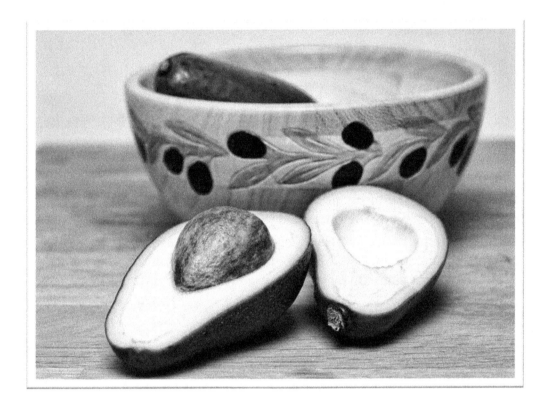

Doctors and dietitians have developed a diet that helps patients with compromised kidney function cut down the amount of waste their body produces, which their kidneys can't filter out. A renal diet is lower in sodium, phosphorus and protein than a typical diet. Every person's body is different, which means that what works for one person may not work for another. Some people have to cut their levels of potassium and calcium as well. A renal diet must be tailored to meet the individual needs and toxin levels of the patient. Keeping a food journal may become necessary and is highly recommended. Sometimes, it can be hard to keep track of all the foods and their amounts; a journal can make keeping track a lot less intimidating. A physical notebook or even a cell phone application can be used for this.

Sodium (mg)

Sodium and table salt are two different components. Table salt is comprised of sodium and chloride. However, sodium by itself is a mineral that is naturally occurring in most of the foods we eat. This is the reason why processed foods are not recommended for someone with kidney problems, or someone who is on a renal diet, due to the added salt that is put into them. Sodium is one of three major electrolytes that help control the fluids going in and out of the cells and tissues in the body. Sodium is responsible for helping control blood pressure and volume, muscle contraction and nerve functions, regulating the acid and base balance of the blood, and balancing the elimination and retention of fluid in the body.

Renal patients are required to monitor their sodium intake because when the kidney's functions become compromised, it is harder for the body to eliminate fluids and excess sodium. The side effects of excess sodium include:

- Increased thirst.
- Edema
- High blood pressure.
- Shortness of breath from fluid being retained in the lungs.
- Heart failure from an overworked and weak heart, which is being forced by the body to work harder.

Limiting sodium can be easier than you think. Since sodium content is always listed on food labels, it is important to get into the habit of checking not only sodium content, but the single serving size as well. As a rule of thumb, fresh is better. Packaged foods typically have added salt, so stick with things that have no salt added to them.

Start comparing the items you use. If it is a spice, steer clear of anything with "salt" in the title. When you are cooking in your home, do not add extra salt to your food under any circumstance. Too much sodium can make chronic kidney disease progress much faster.

Potassium (mg)

Potassium is another one of the three major electrolytes in the body. It is a naturally occurring mineral found in many foods, and in our own bodies. Potassium helps keep our hearts beating regularly and our muscles working correctly. The kidneys have a duty when regulating the amount of potassium in the body. These organs, when healthy, know just how much potassium your body needs. Excess potassium is cleansed from the body through the body's urine output. When you have chronic kidney disease, this naturally occurring regulation in the body becomes compromised. Hyperkalemia (caused by excess potassium), comes with the following symptoms:

- Weakness in the muscles.
- Irregular heartbeat.
- A pulse that is slower than normal.
- Heart attack / Stroke.
- Death

Learning how to limit potassium, just like sodium, is an important part of your renal diet. Foods like bananas, fish, spinach, avocados and potatoes are high in potassium and are foods to avoid. Cut down on your milk and dairy consumption to eight ounces per day. Make sure to read the labels and adhere to the single serving size of the foods you are eating.

Phosphorus (mg)

Phosphorus is a mineral that aids the bones and the muscles in the body. When food is ingested, the small intestines absorb the amount of phosphorus needed for the bones, but the kidneys are in charge of removing the extra phosphorus. When the kidneys can't expel the extra phosphorus, it builds up in the blood and pulls calcium from the bones, making them weak. High amounts of phosphorus can also cause calcium deposits to build up in the heart, lungs, eyes and blood vessels.

Keeping phosphorus levels low, just like sodium and potassium, are important in a renal diet. Stop eating foods that are rich in phosphorus like soda, cheese, meat, milk and seeds. It may be necessary to discuss using phosphate binders with your doctor to keep your levels under control. Make sure to avoid foods with added phosphorus. These will be labeled with "PHOS" on the label.

Protein (g)

Protein levels can be a tricky thing to control if you have chronic kidney disease. Different stages of CKD tolerate protein levels differently, and depending on the stage of CKD, your diet will reflect different level of proteins allowed. Proteins are important to the body, so you can't eliminate them from your diet. You can be aware of your intake, and what your body can or cannot tolerate.

Fluid

It is important for fluid intake to be strictly monitored due to the probability of fluid being retained in the body. When a person is on dialysis, their urine output is decreased, so extra fluid can cause unnecessary strain on the body. Fluid intake levels can be calculated by a nutritionist or doctor on a personal basis. Never drink more than what the doctor tells you is okay, and do not forget to consider solids that turn to liquid at room temperature, or those that are used in cooking.

CHAPTER 8:

Shopping List

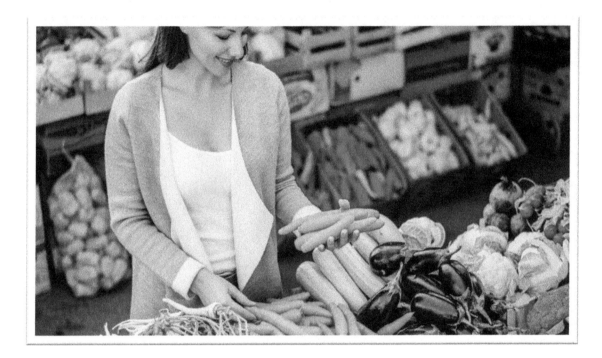

Meat and Meat Substitutes
- Beef
- Chicken
- Eggs
- Egg substitute
- Fish
- Lamb
- Pork, chops / roast
- Tofu
- Tuna (canned)
- Turkey
- Veal

Vegetables
- Arugula
- Bean sprouts
- Cabbage (green/red)
- Carrots
- Cauliflower
- Celery
- Chiles
- Chives
- Coleslaw
- Corn
- Cucumber
- Eggplant
- Endive
- Ginger root
- Green beans
- Lettuce
- Onions
- Parsley
- Radishes
- Turnips
- Vegetables (mixed)
- Water chestnuts (canned)
- Asparagus
- Beets (canned)

Fruits
- Apples
- Blackberries
- Cherries
- Cranberries
- Figs (fresh)
- Fruit cocktail
- Grapefruit
- Grapes
- Lemon
- Lime
- Peaches
- Pear
- Pineapple
- Plums
- Raspberries
- Strawberries
- Tangerines
- Watermelon

Bread and Cereals
- Bagels (plain/blueberry)
- Bread (white/French/Italian)
- Cereals (Kellogg's Corn Flakes, Cheerios, Corn Chex)
- Couscous
- Crackers (unsalted)
- Dinner rolls
- English muffins

Pasta
- Melba toast
- Rice (brown/white)
- Noodles
- Oyster crackers
- Pita bread
- Tortillas
- Pretzels (unsalted)
- Spaghetti

Fats
- Butter
- Cream cheese
- Margarine
- Mayonnaise
- Miracle Whip
- Non-dairy creamers
- Olive oil

Sweets
- Animal crackers
- Angel food cake
- Candy corn
- Chewing gum
- Cotton candy
- Crispy rice treats
- Graham crackers
- Gumdrops
- Gummy bears
- Hard candy
- Hot Tamales candy
- Jell-O
- Jellybeans
- Jolly Rancher
- Lemon cake
- Life Savers

- Marshmallows
- Pie
- Pound cake
- Rice cakes
- Vanilla wafers

Beverages
- 7UP
- Coffee
- Cream soda
- Fruit punch
- Ginger ale
- Grape soda
- Hi-C
- Lemon-lime soda
- Lemonade
- Orange soda
- Root beer
- Tea

Dairy
- Almond milk
- Coffee-mate
- Mocha Mix
- Rice Dream
- Rich's Coffee

Other
- Apple butter
- Corn syrup
- Honey
- Jam
- Jelly
- Maple syrup
- Sugar (powdered, brown or white)

CHAPTER 9:

Breakfast Recipes

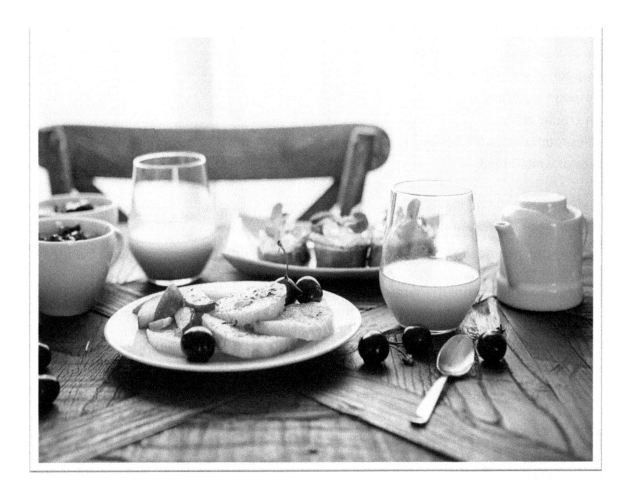

Spiced French Toast

Preparation Time: 15 minutes
Cooking Time: 12 minutes
Servings: 4

Ingredients:
4 eggs
½ cup of Homemade Rice Milk (you may use unsweetened store-bought) or almond milk.
¼ cup of freshly squeezed orange juice.
1 teaspoon of ground cinnamon.
½ teaspoon of ground ginger.
Pinch ground cloves.
1 tablespoon of unsalted butter (divided).
8 slices of white bread.

Directions:

- Whisk eggs, rice milk, orange juice, cinnamon, ginger and cloves until well blended in a large bowl.
- Melt half the butter in a large skillet. It should be in medium-high heat only.
- Drench four of the bread slices in the egg mixture until well soaked, and place them in the skillet.
- Cook the toast until golden brown on both sides, turning once, about 6 minutes total.
- Repeat with the remaining butter and bread.
- Serve 2 pieces of hot French toast to each person.

Nutrition:
Calories - 236;
Total fat - 11g;
Saturated fat - 4g;
Cholesterol - 220mg;
Sodium - 84mg;
Carbohydrates - 27g;
 Fiber - 1g;
Phosphorus - 119mg;
Potassium - 158mg;
Protein - 11g

Breakfast Tacos

Preparation Time: 10 minutes

Cooking Time: 10 minutes

Servings: 4

Ingredients:

1 teaspoon of olive oil

½ sweet onions (chopped)

½ red bell pepper (chopped)

½ teaspoon of minced garlic

4 eggs (beaten)

½ teaspoon of ground cumin

Pinch red pepper flakes

4 tortillas

¼ cup of tomato salsa

Directions:

- ➢ Heat the oil in a large skillet in a medium heat only.
- ➢ Add the onion, bell pepper, garlic and sauté until softened after about 5 minutes.
- ➢ Add the eggs, cumin and red pepper flakes; then scramble the eggs with the vegetables until cooked through and fluffy.
- ➢ Spoon one-fourth of the egg mixture into the center of each tortilla, and top each with 1 tablespoon of salsa.
- ➢ Serve immediately.

Nutrition:

Calories - 211;

Total fat - 7g;

Saturated fat - 2g;

Cholesterol - 211mg;

Sodium - 346mg;

Carbohydrates - 17g;

Fiber - 1g;

Phosphorus - 120mg;

Potassium - 141mg;

Protein - 9g

Pineapple Sorbet Smoothie

Preparation Time: 5 minutes

Cooking Time: 0 minutes

Servings: 1

Ingredients:

¾ cup of pineapple sorbet

1 scoop of protein powder

½ cup of water

2 ice cubes (optional)

Directions:

➢ First, begin by putting everything into a blender jug.

➢ Pulse it for 30 seconds until well blended.

➢ Serve chilled.

Nutrition:

Calories - 180

Total Fat - 1g

Saturated Fat - 0.5g

Cholesterol - 40mg

Sodium - 86mg

Carbohydrate - 30.5g

Dietary Fiber - 0g

Sugars - 28g

Protein - 13g

Calcium - 9mg

Phosphorous - 164mg

Potassium - 111mg

Vanilla Fruit Smoothie

Preparation Time: 5 minutes

Cooking Time: 0 minutes

Servings: 2

Ingredients:

2 oz. of mango (peeled and cubed)

2 oz. of strawberries

2 oz. of avocado flesh (cubed)

2 oz. of banana (peeled)

2 scoops of protein powder

1 cup of cold water

1 cup of crushed ice

Directions:

> ➢ First, begin by putting everything into a blender jug.
> ➢ Pulse it for 30 seconds until well blended.
> ➢ Serve chilled.

Nutrition:

Calories - 228

Total Fat - 7.6g

Saturated Fat - 2.1g

Cholesterol - 65mg

Sodium - 58mg

Total Carbohydrate - 19g

Dietary Fiber - 3.6g

Sugars - 9.8g

Protein - 23.4g

Calcium - 112mg

Phosphorous - 216 mg

Potassium - 504mg

Protein Berry Smoothie

Preparation Time: 5 minutes

Cooking Time: 0 minutes

Servings: 2

Ingredients:

4 oz. of water

1 cup of frozen mixed berries

2 ice cubes

1 teaspoon of blueberry essence

2 scoops of whey protein powder

Directions:

➢ First, begin by putting everything into a blender jug.
➢ Pulse it for 30 seconds until well blended.
➢ Serve chilled.

Nutrition:

Calories - 248

Total Fat - 11.4g

Saturated Fat - 6.7g

Cholesterol - 98mg

Sodium - 67mg

Carbohydrate - 13.3g

Dietary Fiber - 2.5g

Sugars - 6.1g

Protein - 23.3g

Calcium - 132mg

Phosphorous - 152mg

Potassium - 296mg

Power-Boosting Smoothie

Preparation Time: 5 minutes

Cooking Time: 0 minutes

Servings: 2

Ingredients:

½ cup of water

½ cup of non-dairy whipped topping

2 scoops of whey protein powder

1½ cups of frozen blueberries

Directions:

➢ In a high-speed blender, add all ingredients and pulse till smooth.

➢ Transfer into 2 serving glass and serve immediately.

Nutrition:

Calories - 242

Fat - 7g

Carbs - 23.8g

Protein - 23.2g

Potassium (K) - 263mg

Sodium (Na) - 63mg

Phosphorous - 30 mg

Distinctive Pineapple Smoothie

Preparation Time: 5 minutes

Cooking Time: 0 minutes

Servings: 2

Ingredients:

¼ cup of crushed ice cubes

2 scoops of vanilla whey protein powder

1 cup of water

1½ cups of pineapple

Directions:

➢ In a high-speed blender, add all ingredients and pulse till smooth.
➢ Transfer into 2 serving glass and serve immediately.

Nutrition:

Calories - 117

Fat - 2.1g

Carbs - 18.2g

Protein - 22.7g

Potassium (K) - 296mg

Sodium (Na) - 81mg

Phosphorous - 28 mg

Apple Pumpkin Muffins

Preparation Time: 15 minutes

Cooking Time: 20 minutes

Servings: 12

Ingredients:

1 cup of all-purpose flour

1 cup of wheat bran

2 teaspoons of Phosphorus Powder

1 cup of pumpkin purée

¼ cup of honey

¼ cup of olive oil

1 egg

1 teaspoon of vanilla extract

½ cup of cored diced apple

Directions:

➢ Preheat the oven to 400°F.

➢ Line 12 muffin cups with paper liners.

➢ Stir together the flour, wheat bran and baking powder. Mix this in a medium bowl.

➢ In a small bowl, whisk together the pumpkin, honey, olive oil, egg and vanilla.

➢ Stir the pumpkin mixture into the flour mixture until just combined.

➢ Stir in the diced apple.

➢ Spoon the batter in the muffin cups.

➢ Bake for about 20 minutes, or until a toothpick inserted in the center of a muffin comes out clean.

Nutrition (1 muffin):

Calories - 125;

Total Fat - 5g;

Saturated Fat - 1g;

Cholesterol - 18mg;

Sodium - 8mg;

Carbohydrates - 20g;

Fiber - 3g;

Phosphorus - 120mg;

Potassium - 177mg;

Protein - 2g

Mexican Scrambled Eggs in Tortilla

Preparation Time: 5 minutes

Cooking Time: 2 minutes

Servings: 2

Ingredients:

2 medium corn tortillas

4 egg whites

1 teaspoon of cumin

3 teaspoons of green chilies (diced)

½ teaspoon of hot pepper sauce

2 tablespoons of salsa

½ teaspoon of salt

Directions:

➢ Spray some cooking spray on a medium skillet and heat for a few seconds.
➢ Whisk the eggs with the green chilies, hot sauce and comminute
➢ Add the eggs into the pan, and whisk with a spatula to scramble. Then, add salt.
➢ Cook until fluffy and done (1-2 minutes) over low heat.
➢ Open the tortillas and spread 1 tablespoon of salsa on each.
➢ Distribute the egg mixture onto the tortillas and wrap gently to make a burrito.
➢ Serve warm.

Nutrition:

Calories - 44.1 kcal

Carbohydrate - 2.23 g

Protein - 7.69 g

Sodium - 854 mg

Potassium - 189 mg

Phosphorus - 22 mg

Dietary Fiber - 0.5 g

Fat - 0.39 g

Raspberry Smoothie

Preparation Time: 5 minutes

Cooking Time: 0 minutes

Servings: 2

Ingredients:

1 cup frozen of raspberries

1 medium peach (pitted, sliced)

½ cup of tofu

1 tablespoon of honey

1 cup of milk

Directions:

➢ First, begin by putting everything into a blender jug.

➢ Pulse it for 30 seconds until well blended.

➢ Serve chilled.

Nutrition:

Calories - 223

Total Fat - 2.7g

Saturated Fat - 0.3g

Cholesterol - 0mg

Sodium - 99mg

Carbohydrate - 49.9g

Dietary Fiber - 7.2g

Sugars - 43.1g

Protein - 3.6g

Calcium - 176mg

Phosphorous - 95mg

Potassium - 426mg

Citrus Pineapple Shake

Preparation Time: 5 minutes

Cooking Time: 0 minutes

Servings: 2

Ingredients:

½ cup of pineapple juice

½ cup of almond milk

1 cup of orange sherbet

½ cup of egg (pasteurized)

Directions:

➤ Pour the almond milk, pineapple juice, sherbet and egg into the blender.

➤ Blend well for 1 minute then refrigerate to chill.

➤ Serve.

Nutrition:

Calories - 242

Total Fat - 8.2g

Saturated Fat - 2.8g

Cholesterol - 227mg

Sodium - 155mg

Carbohydrate - 33g

Dietary Fiber - 1.1g

Sugars - 26.2g

Protein - 8.9g

Calcium - 80mg

Phosphorous - 121mg

Potassium - 234mg

Pineapple Smoothie

Preparation Time: 5 minutes

Cooking Time: 0 minutes

Servings: 2

Ingredients:

¾ cup of pineapple sherbet

1 scoop of protein powder

½ cup of water

2 ice cubes

Directions:

➢ Add the water, pineapple sherbet, protein powder and ice to a blender.

➢ Blend the pineapple smoothie for 1 minute.

➢ Serve.

Nutrition:

Calories - 91

Total Fat - 0.6g

Saturated Fat - 0.2g

Cholesterol - 7mg

Sodium - 36mg

Carbohydrate - 10.4g

Dietary Fiber - 0g

Sugars - 8g

Protein - 11.9g

Calcium - 208mg

Phosphorous - 49mg

Potassium - 25mg

American Blueberry Pancakes

Preparation Time: 5 minutes

Cooking Time: 10 minutes

Servings: 6

Ingredients:

1 ½ cups of all-purpose flour, sifted

1 cup of buttermilk

3 tablespoons of sugar

2 tablespoons of unsalted butter (melted)

2 teaspoons of baking powder

2 eggs (beaten)

1 cup of canned blueberries (rinsed)

Directions:

- ➢ Combine the baking powder, flour and sugar in a bowl.
- ➢ Make a hole in the center and slowly add the rest of the ingredients.
- ➢ Begin to stir gently from the sides to the center with a spatula, until you get a smooth and creamy batter.
- ➢ With cooking spray, spray the pan and place over medium heat.
- ➢ Take one measuring cup and fill ⅓rd of its capacity with the batter to make each pancake.
- ➢ Use a spoon to pour the pancake batter and let cook until golden brown. Flip once to cook the other side.
- ➢ Serve warm with optional agave syrup.

Nutrition:

Calories - 251.69 kcal

Carbohydrate - 41.68 g

Protein - 7.2 g

Sodium - 186.68 mg

Potassium - 142.87 mg

Phosphorus - 255.39 mg

Dietary Fiber - 1.9 g

Fat - 6.47 g

Raspberry Peach Breakfast Smoothie

Preparation Time: 5 minutes

Cooking Time: 1 minute

Servings: 2

Ingredients:

⅓ cup of raspberries (it can be frozen)

½ peach (skin and pit removed)

1 tablespoon of honey

1 cup of coconut water

Directions:

➢ Mix all ingredients together and blend it until smooth.

➢ Pour and serve chilled in a tall glass or mason jar.

Nutrition:

Calories - 86.3 kcal

Carbohydrate - 20.6 g

Protein - 1.4 g

Sodium - 3 mg

Potassium - 109 mg

Phosphorus - 36.08 mg

Dietary Fiber - 2.6 g

Fat - 0.31 g

Mango Lassi Smoothie

Preparation Time: 5 minutes

Cooking Time: 0 minute

Servings: 2

Ingredients:

½ cup of plain yogurt

½ cup of plain water

½ cup of sliced mango

1 tablespoon of sugar

¼ teaspoon of cardamom

¼ teaspoon cinnamon

¼ cup of lime juice

Directions:

> ➢ Pulse all the above ingredients in a blender until smooth (around 1 minute).
> ➢ Pour into tall glasses or mason jars and serve chilled immediately.

Nutrition:

Calories - 89.02 kcal

Carbohydrate - 14.31 g

Protein - 2.54 g

Sodium - 30 mg

Potassium - 185.67 mg

Phosphorus - 67.88 mg

Dietary Fiber - 0.77 g

Fat - 2.05 g

Breakfast Maple Sausage

Preparation Time: 15 minutes

Cooking Time: 8 minutes

Servings: 12

Ingredients:

1 pound of pork (minced)

½ pound of lean turkey meat (ground)

¼ teaspoon of nutmeg

½ teaspoon of black pepper

¼ all spice

2 tablespoons of maple syrup

1 tablespoon of water

Directions:

➢ Combine all the ingredients in a bowl.
➢ Cover and refrigerate for 3-4 hours.
➢ Take the mixture and form into small flat patties with your hand (around 10 to 12 patties).
➢ Lightly grease a medium skillet with oil and shallow fry the patties over medium to high heat, until brown (around 4-5 minutes on each side).
➢ Serve hot.

Nutrition:

Calories - 53.85 kcal

Carbohydrate - 2.42 g

Protein - 8.5 g

Sodium - 30.96 mg

Potassium - 84.68 mg

Phosphorus - 83.49 mg

Dietary Fiber - 0.03 g

Fat - 0.9 g

Summer Veggie Omelet

Preparation Time: 5 minutes

Cooking Time: 5 minutes

Servings: 2

Ingredients:

4 large egg whites

¼ cup of sweet corn (frozen)

⅓ cup of zucchini (grated)

2 green onions (sliced)

1 tablespoon of cream cheese

Kosher pepper

Directions:

➢ Grease a medium pan with some cooking spray and add the onions, corn and grated zucchini.

➢ Sauté for a couple of minutes until softened.

➢ Beat the eggs together with the water, cream cheese and pepper in a bowl.

➢ Add the eggs into the veggie mixture in the pan and let cook while moving the edges from inside to outside with a spatula, to allow raw egg to cook through the edges.

➢ Turn the omelet with the aid of a dish (placed over the pan and flipped upside down and then back to the pan).

➢ Let sit for another 1 to 2 minutes.

➢ Fold in half and serve.

Nutrition:

Calories - 90 kcal

Carbohydrate - 15.97 g

Protein - 8.07 g

Sodium - 227 mg

Potassium - 244.24 mg

Phosphorus - 45.32 mg

Dietary Fiber - 0.88 g

Fat - 2.44 g

Raspberry Overnight Porridge

Preparation Time: Overnight

Cooking Time: 0 minute

Servings: 12

Ingredients:

⅓ cup of rolled oats

½ cup of almond milk

1 tablespoon of honey

5-6 raspberries (fresh or canned, and unsweetened)

Directions:

➢ Combine the oats, almond milk and honey in a mason jar and place into the fridge for overnight.

➢ Serve the next morning with the raspberries on top.

Nutrition:

Calories - 143.6 kcal

Carbohydrate - 34.62 g

Protein - 3.44 g

Sodium - 77.88 mg

Potassium - 153¼ mg

Phosphorus - 99.3 mg

Dietary Fiber - 7.56 g

Fat - 3.91 g

Turkey and Spinach Scramble on Melba Toast

Preparation Time: 2 minutes

Cooking Time: 15 minutes

Servings: 2

Ingredients:

1 teaspoon of Extra virgin olive oil

1 cup of Raw spinach

½ clove of Garlic (minced)

1 teaspoon of Nutmeg (grated)

1 cup of Cooked and diced turkey breast

4 slices of Melba toast

1 teaspoon of Balsamic vinegar

Directions:

➢ Heat a pot over a source of heat and add oil.
➢ Add turkey and heat through for 6 to 8 minutes.
➢ Add spinach, garlic and nutmeg. Then, stir-fry for 6 minutes more.
➢ Plate up the Melba toast and top with spinach and turkey scramble.
➢ Drizzle with balsamic vinegar and serve.

Nutrition:

Calories - 301

Fat - 19g

Carbs - 12g

Phosphorus - 215mg

Potassium - 269mg

Sodium - 360mg

Protein - 19g

Vegetable Omelet

Preparation Time: 15 minutes

Cooking Time: 10 minutes

Servings: 3

Ingredients:

4 Egg whites

1 Egg

2 Tablespoons of chopped fresh parsley

2 Tablespoons of water

Olive oil spray

½ cup of chopped and boiled red bell pepper

¼ cup of chopped scallion (both green and white parts)

Ground black pepper

Directions:

➢ Whisk together the egg, egg whites, parsley and water until well blended. Then, set it aside.

➢ Spray a skillet with olive oil spray and place over medium heat.

➢ Sauté the peppers and scallion for 3 minutes or until softened.

➢ Over the vegetables, you can now pour the egg and cook, swirling the skillet for 2 minutes or until the edges start to set. Cook until set.

➢ Season with black pepper and serve.

Nutrition:

Calories - 77

Fat - 3g

Carbs - 2g

Phosphorus - 67mg

Potassium - 194mg

Sodium - 229mg

Protein - 12g

Cinnamon Egg Smoothie

Preparation Time: 8 minutes

Cooking Time: 0 minutes

Servings: 2

Ingredients:

½ teaspoon of ground cinnamon

1 teaspoon of stevia

⅛ teaspoon of vanilla extract

8 oz. of egg white (pasteurized)

3 tablespoons of whipped topping

Directions:

 ➢ Mix the stevia, egg whites, cinnamon and vanilla in a mixer.
 ➢ Serve with whipped topping.

Nutrition:

Calories - 95

Total Fat - 1.2g

Saturated Fat - 0.6g

Cholesterol - 3mg

Sodium - 120mg

Carbohydrate - 3.1g

Dietary Fiber - 0.3g

Sugars - 0.8g

Protein - 12.5g

Calcium - 18mg

Phosphorous - 185mg

Potassium - 194mg

Protein Peach Smoothie

Preparation Time: 5 minutes

Cooking Time: 0 minutes

Servings: 1

Ingredients:

½ cup of ice

2 tablespoons of egg whites (pasteurized)

¾ cup of fresh peaches

1 teaspoon of stevia

Directions:

➢ First, begin by putting everything into a blender jug.
➢ Pulse it for 30 seconds until well blended.
➢ Serve chilled.

Nutrition:

Calories - 195

Total Fat - 0.3g

Saturated Fat - 0g

Cholesterol - 0mg

Sodium - 347mg

Carbohydrate - 17g

Dietary Fiber - 1.7g

Sugars - 14.2g

Protein - 24.1g

Calcium - 25mg

Phosphorous - 233mg

Potassium - 526mg

Cranberry Cucumber Smoothie

Preparation Time: 5 minutes

Cooking Time: 0 minutes

Servings: 1

Ingredients:

1 cup of frozen cranberries

1 medium cucumber (peeled and sliced)

1 stalk of celery

1 teaspoon of lime juice

Directions:

➢ First, begin by putting everything into a blender jug.

➢ Pulse it for 30 seconds until well blended.

➢ Serve chilled.

Nutrition:

Calories - 119

Total Fat - 0.4g

Saturated Fat - 0.1g

Cholesterol - 0mg

Sodium - 21mg

Carbohydrate - 25.1g

Dietary Fiber - 6g

Sugars - 10g

Protein - 2.3g

Calcium - 79mg

Phosphorous - 184mg

Potassium - 325mg

Mexican Style Burritos

Preparation Time: 5 minutes

Cooking Time: 15 minutes

Servings: 2

Ingredients:

1 Tablespoon of olive oil

2 Corn tortillas

¼ cup of red onions (chopped)

¼ cup of red bell peppers (chopped)

½ Red chili (deseeded and chopped)

2 Eggs

Juice from 1 lime

1 Tablespoon of Cilantro (chopped)

Directions:

➢ Turn the broiler to medium heat and place the tortillas underneath for 1 to 2 minutes on each side or until lightly toasted.

➢ Remove and keep the broiler on.

➢ Sauté onion, chili and bell peppers for 5 to 6 minutes or until soft.

➢ Place the eggs on top of the onions and peppers. Then, place skillet under the broiler for 5 to 6 minutes, or until the eggs are cooked.

➢ Serve half the eggs and vegetables on top of each tortilla and sprinkle with cilantro and lime juice to serve.

Nutrition:

Calories - 202

Fat - 13g

Carbs - 19g

Phosphorus - 184mg

Potassium - 233mg

Sodium - 77mg

Protein - 9g

CHAPTER 10:

Lunch Recipes

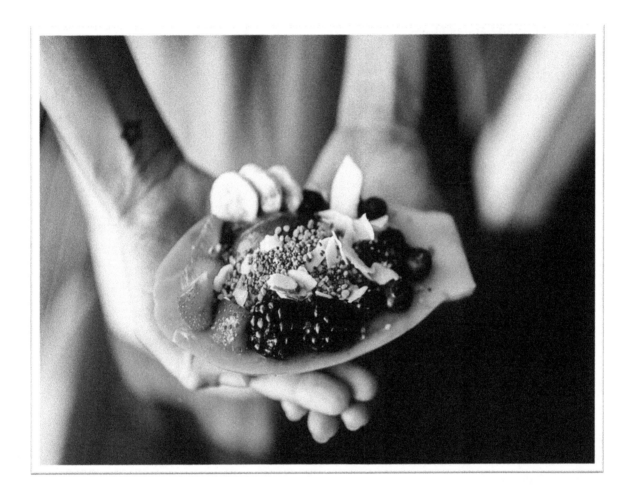

Tilapia with Lemon Garlic Sauce

Preparation Time: 15 minutes

Cooking Time: 30 minutes

Servings: 4

Ingredients:

Pepper

1 teaspoon of dried parsley flakes

1 clove of garlic (finely chopped)

1 tablespoon of butter (melted)

3 tablespoons of fresh lemon juice

4 tilapia fillets

Directions:

➢ First, spray bake dish with non-stick cooking spray; then preheat oven at 375 degrees Fahrenheit (190oC).
➢ In cool water, rinse tilapia fillets. Then, pat dry the fillets using paper towels.
➢ Place tilapia fillets in the baking dish; then pour butter and lemon juice, and top off with pepper, parsley and garlic.
➢ Bake tilapia in the preheated oven for 30 minutes and wait until fish is white.
➢ Enjoy!

Nutrition:

Calories - 168;

Carbs - 4g;

Protein - 24g;

Fats - 5g;

Phosphorus - 207mg;

Potassium - 431mg;

Sodium - 85mg

Spinach with Tuscan White Beans and Shrimps

Preparation Time: 5 minutes

Cooking Time: 15 minutes

Servings: 4

Ingredients:

1 ½ ounces of crumbled reduce-fat feta cheese

5 cups of baby spinach

15 ounces of cannellini beans can (rinsed and drained with no added salt)

½ cup of low sodium, fat-free chicken broth

2 tablespoons of balsamic vinegar

2 teaspoons of chopped fresh sage

4 cloves of garlic (minced)

1 medium onion (chopped)

1-pound large shrimp (peeled and deveined)

2 tablespoons of olive oil

Directions:

➢ Heat 1 teaspoon oil. Heat it over medium-high.

➢ Then, for about 2 to 3 minutes, cook the shrimps using the heated skillet, and place them on a plate.

➢ Heat on the same skillet the sage, garlic and onions. Then, cook for about 4 minutes, add and stir in vinegar for 30 seconds.

➢ For about 2 minutes, add chicken broth. Then, add spinach and beans and cook for an additional 2 to 3 minutes.

➢ Remove skillet then add and stir in cooked shrimps topped with feta cheese.

➢ Serve and divide into 4 bowls.

Nutrition:

Calories - 343

Carbs - 21g

Protein - 22g

Fats - 11g

Phosphorus - 400mg

Potassium - 599mg

Sodium - 766mg

Bagel with Salmon and Egg

Preparation Time: 15 minutes

Cooking Time: 10 minutes

Servings: 1

Ingredients:

Bagel ½

1 tablespoon of cream cheese

1 tablespoon of scallions

½ teaspoon of fresh dill

2 fresh basil leaves

1 slice of tomato

4 pieces of arugula

1 large egg

1 ounce of cooked salmon

Directions:

➢ Start by slicing the bagel through the center horizontally. Take one half of the bagel and toast it in an oven or a toaster.
➢ Finely chop the dill, basil leaves and scallions. Then, set aside.
➢ Add in the cream cheese. Toss in the chopped dill, basil and scallions. Mix well to combine.
➢ Take the toasted bagel and spread the herbs and cream cheese mixture evenly over it.
➢ Place the tomato slice and arugula on top. Then, set aside.
➢ Take a small mixing bowl, and then beat the egg.
➢ Take a non-stick saucepan and grease it using cooking spray. Stir after pouring the beaten egg into the pan and cook for about 1 minute over medium heat. Keep stirring to make a perfect scrambled egg.
➢ Take the cooked salmon and place it in the same pan as the egg. This will help you heat the salmon and cook the egg at the same time.
➢ Place the scrambled egg over the tomato slice and top it with the salmon.

Nutrition:

Protein - 19 g Fat - 14 g

Carbohydrates - 29 g

Cholesterol - 218 mg

Potassium - 338 mg

Sodium - 378 mg

Phosphorus - 270 mg Fiber - 2.6 g Calcium - 77 m

Baked Fish in Cream Sauce

Preparation Time: 10 minutes

Cooking Time: 40 minutes

Servings: 4

Ingredients:

1-pound haddock

½ cup of all-purpose flour

2 tablespoons of butter (unsalted)

¼ teaspoon of pepper

2 cups fat-free nondairy creamer

¼ cup of water

Directions:

- ➤ Preheat your oven to 350 degrees F.
- ➤ Spray baking pan with oil.
- ➤ Sprinkle with a little flour.
- ➤ Arrange fish on the pan.
- ➤ Season with pepper.
- ➤ Sprinkle remaining flour on the fish.
- ➤ Spread creamer on both sides of the fish.
- ➤ Bake for 40 minutes, or until golden.
- ➤ Spread cream sauce on top of the fish before serving.

Nutrition:

Calories - 383

Protein - 24 g

Carbohydrates - 46 g

Fat - 11 g

Cholesterol - 79 mg

Sodium - 253 mg

Potassium - 400 mg

Phosphorus - 266 mg

Calcium - 46 mg

Fiber - 0.4 g

Shrimp in Garlic Sauce

Preparation Time: 10 minutes

Cooking Time: 6 minutes

Servings: 4

Ingredients:

3 tablespoons of butter (unsalted)

¼ cup of onion (minced)

3 cloves of garlic (minced)

1 pound of shrimp (shelled and deveined)

½ cup of half and half creamer

¼ cup of white wine

2 tablespoons of fresh basil

Black pepper to taste

Directions:

➢ Add butter to a pan over medium low heat.

➢ Let it melt.

➢ Add the onion and garlic.

➢ Cook for it 1-2 minutes.

➢ Add the shrimp and cook for 2 minutes.

➢ Transfer shrimp on a serving platter and set aside.

➢ Add the rest of the ingredients.

➢ Let it simmer for 3 minutes.

➢ Pour sauce over the shrimp and serve.

Nutrition:

Calories - 482

Protein - 33 g

Carbohydrates - 46 g

Fat - 11 g

Cholesterol - 230 mg

Sodium - 213 mg

Potassium - 514 mg

Phosphorus - 398 mg

Calcium - 133 mg

Fiber - 2.0 g

Fish Taco

Preparation Time: 40 minutes

Cooking Time: 10 minutes

Servings: 6

Ingredients:

1 tablespoon of lime juice

1 tablespoon of olive oil

1 clove of garlic (minced)

1 pound of cod fillets

½ teaspoon of ground cumin

¼ teaspoon of black pepper

½ teaspoon of chili powder

¼ cup of sour cream

½ cup of mayonnaise

2 tablespoons of non-dairy milk

1 cup of shredded cabbage

½ cup of chopped onion

½ bunch cilantro (chopped)

12 corn tortillas

Directions:

➢ Drizzle lemon juice over the fish fillet.
➢ Then, coat it with olive oil and season with garlic, cumin, pepper and chili powder.
➢ Let it sit for 30 minutes.
➢ Broil fish for 10 minutes, flipping halfway through.
➢ Flake the fish using a fork.
➢ In a bowl, mix sour cream, milk and mayo.
➢ Assemble tacos by filling each tortilla with mayo mixture, cabbage, onion, cilantro and fish flakes.

Nutrition:

Calories – 366 Protein - 18 g

Carbohydrates - 31 g

Fat - 19 g Cholesterol - 40 mg

Sodium - 194 mg Potassium - 507 mg

Phosphorus - 327 mg Calcium - 138 mg Fiber - 4.3 g

Baked Trout

Preparation Time: 5 minutes

Cooking Time: 10 minutes

Servings: 8

Ingredients:

2-pound trout fillet

1 tablespoon of oil

1 teaspoon of salt-free lemon pepper

½ teaspoon of paprika

Directions:

- ➢ Preheat your oven to 350 degrees F.
- ➢ Coat fillet with oil.
- ➢ Place fish on a baking pan.
- ➢ Season with lemon pepper and paprika.
- ➢ Bake for 10 minutes.

Nutrition:

Calories - 161

Protein - 21 g

Carbohydrates - 0 g

Fat - 8 g

Cholesterol - 58 mg

Sodium - 109 mg

Potassium - 385 mg

Phosphorus - 227 mg

Calcium - 75 mg

Fiber - 0.1 g

Fish with Mushrooms

Preparation Time: 5 minutes

Cooking Time: 16 minutes

Servings: 4

Ingredients:

1 pound cod fillet

2 tablespoons of butter

¼ cup of chopped white onion

1 cup of fresh mushrooms

1 teaspoon of dried thyme

Directions:

- ➢ Put the fish in a baking pan.
- ➢ Preheat your oven to 450 degrees F.
- ➢ Melt the butter and cook the onion and mushroom for 1 minute.
- ➢ Spread mushroom mixture on top of the fish.
- ➢ Season with thyme.
- ➢ Bake in the oven for 15 minutes.

Nutrition:

Calories - 156

Protein - 21 g

Carbohydrates - 3 g

Fat - 7 g

Cholesterol - 49 mg

Sodium - 110 mg

Potassium - 561 mg

Phosphorus - 225 mg

Calcium - 30 mg

Fiber - 0.5 g

Roasted Veggies Mediterranean Style

Preparation Time: 5 minutes

Cooking Time: 10 minutes

Servings: 2

Ingredients:

½ teaspoon of freshly grated lemon zest

1 cup of grape tomatoes

1 tablespoon of extra-virgin olive oil

1 tablespoon of lemon juice

1 teaspoon of dried oregano

10 pitted black olives (sliced)

12-ounce broccoli crowns, trimmed and cut into bite-sized pieces

2 cloves of garlic (minced)

2 teaspoons of capers (rinsed)

Directions:

➢ Preheat oven to 350oF and grease a baking sheet with cooking spray.
➢ In a large bowl, toss salt, garlic, oil, tomatoes and broccoli together until thoroughly coated.
➢ Spread broccoli on prepped baking sheet and bake for 8 to 10 minutes.
➢ In another large bowl, mix capers, oregano, olives, lemon juice, and lemon zest. Mix in roasted vegetables and serve while still warm.

Nutrition:

Calories - 110

Carbs - 16g

Protein - 6g

Fats - 4g

Phosphorus - 138mg

Potassium - 745mg

Sodium - 214mg

Chicken Meatloaf with Veggies

Preparation Time: 20 minutes

Cooking Time: 1-1¼ hours

Servings: 4

Ingredients (for meatloaf):

½ cup of cooked chickpeas

2 egg whites

2½ teaspoons of poultry seasoning

Salt and freshly ground black pepper, to taste

10-ounce lean ground chicken

1 cup of red bell pepper (seeded and minced)

1 cup of celery stalk (minced)

⅓ cup of steel-cut oats

1 cup of tomato puree (divided)

2 tablespoons of dried onion flakes (crushed)

1 tablespoon of prepared mustard

Ingredients (for veggies):

2 pounds of summer squash (sliced)

16-ounce of frozen Brussels sprouts

2 tablespoons of extra-virgin olive oil

Salt and freshly ground black pepper, to taste

Directions:

➢ Preheat the oven to 350 degrees F. Grease a 9x5-inch loaf pan.
➢ In a mixer, add chickpeas, egg whites, poultry seasoning, salt and black pepper. Then, pulse till smooth.
➢ Transfer a combination in a large bowl.
➢ Add chicken, veggies oats, ½ cup of tomato puree and onion flakes. Then, mix till well combined.
➢ Transfer the amalgamation into prepared loaf pan evenly.
➢ With both hands, press, down the amalgamation slightly.
➢ In another bowl, mix together mustard and the remaining tomato puree.
➢ Place the mustard mixture over loaf pan evenly.
➢ Bake approximately 1-1¼ hours or till desired doneness.
➢ Meanwhile, in a big pan of water, arrange a steamer basket.
➢ Bring to a boil and set summer time squash I steamer basket.
➢ Cover and steam for approximately 10 to 12 minutes.
➢ Drain well and aside.
➢ Now, prepare the Brussels sprouts according to package's directions.
➢ In a big bowl, add veggies, oil, salt and black pepper. Then, toss to coat well.
➢ Serve the meatloaf with veggies.

Nutrition:

Calories - 420

Fat - 9g

Carbohydrates - 21g

Fiber - 14g

Protein - 36g

Phosphorus - 431 mg

Potassium - 472 mg

Sodium - 249 mg

Roasted Spatchcock Chicken

Preparation Time: twenty or so minutes

Cooking Time: 50 minutes

Servings: 4 to 6

Ingredients:

1 (4-pound) whole chicken

1 (1-inch) piece of fresh ginger (sliced)

4 garlic cloves (chopped)

1 small bunch of fresh thyme

Pinch of cayenne

Salt and freshly ground black pepper

¼ cup of fresh lemon juice

3 tablespoons of extra virgin olive oil

Directions:

➢ Arrange chicken, breast side down, onto a large cutting board.

➢ With a kitchen shear, begin with thigh and cut along one side of backbone and turn chicken around.

➢ Now, cut along sleep issues and discard the backbone.

➢ Change the inside and open it like a book.

➢ Flatten the backbone firmly to flatten.

➢ In a food processor, add all ingredients except chicken, and pulse till smooth.

➢ In a big baking dish, add the marinade mixture.

➢ Add chicken and coat with marinade generously.

➢ With a plastic wrap, cover the baking dish and refrigerate to marinate for overnight.

➢ Preheat the oven to 450 degrees F. Arrange a rack in a roasting pan.

➢ Remove the chicken from refrigerator make onto rack over roasting pan, skin side down.

➢ Roast for about 50 minutes, turning once in the middle way.

Nutrition:

Calories - 419

Fat - 14g

Carbohydrates - 28g

Fiber - 4g

Protein - 40g

Phosphorus - 281 mg

Potassium - 354 mg

Sodium - 165 mg

Herbs and Lemony Roasted Chicken

Preparation Time: 15 minutes

Cooking Time: 1 ½ hours

Servings: 8

Ingredients:

½ teaspoon of ground black pepper

½ teaspoon of mustard powder

½ teaspoon of salt

1 3-lb whole chicken

1 teaspoon of garlic powder

2 lemons

2 tablespoons of olive oil

2 teaspoons of Italian seasoning

Directions:

➤ In small bowl, thoroughly mix black pepper, garlic powder, mustard powder and salt.
➤ Rinse chicken well and slice off giblets.
➤ In a greased 9 x 13 baking dish, place chicken and add 1 ½ teaspoons of seasoning made earlier inside the chicken, and rub the remaining seasoning around chicken.
➤ In small bowl, mix olive oil and juice from 2 lemons. Drizzle over chicken.
➤ Bake chicken in a preheated 350oF oven until juices run clear, after about 1 ½ hours.
➤ Every once in a while, paste chicken with its juices.

Nutrition:

Calories - 190

Carbs - 2g

Protein - 35g

Fats - 9g

Phosphorus - 341mg

Potassium - 439mg

Sodium - 328mg

Mouthwatering Beef and Chili Stew

Preparation Time: 15 minutes

Cooking Time: 7 hours

Servings: 6

Ingredients:

½ medium red onion, thinly sliced into half moons

½ tablespoon of vegetable oil

10ounce of flat cut beef brisket (whole)

½ cup of low sodium stock

¾ cup of water

½ tablespoon of honey

½ tablespoon of chili powder

½ teaspoon of smoked paprika

½ teaspoon of dried thyme

1 teaspoon of black pepper

1 tablespoon of corn starch

Directions:

➢ Throw the sliced onion into the slow cooker first.
➢ Add a splash of oil to a large hot skillet and briefly seal the beef on all sides.
➢ Remove the beef from skillet and place in the slow cooker.
➢ Add the stock, water, honey and spices to the same skillet that you cooked the beef in.
➢ Loosen the browned bits from bottom of pan with spatula. (Hint: These brown bits at the bottom are called the fond.)
➢ Allow juice to simmer until the volume is reduced by about half.
➢ Pour the juice over beef in the slow cooker.
➢ Set slow cooker on Low and cook for approximately 7 hours.
➢ Take the beef out of the slow cooker and onto a platter.
➢ Shred it with two forks.
➢ Pour the remaining juice into a medium saucepan. Bring to a simmer.
➢ Whisk the cornstarch with two tablespoons of water.
➢ Add to the juice and cook until slightly thickened.
➢ For a thicker sauce, simmer and reduce the juice a bit more before adding cornstarch.
➢ Pour the sauce over the meat and serve.

Nutrition:

Calories – 128 Protein - 13g Carbohydrates - 6g

Fat - 6g Cholesterol - 39mg Sodium - 228mg Potassium - 202mg

Phosphorus - 119mg Calcium - 16mg Fiber - 1g

Beef and Three Pepper Stew

Preparation Time: 15 minutes

Cooking Time: 6 hours

Servings: 6

Ingredients:

10ounce of flat cut beef brisket (whole)

1 teaspoon of dried thyme

1 teaspoon of black pepper

1 clove of garlic

½ cup of green onion (thinly sliced)

½ cup of low sodium chicken stock

2 cups of water

1 large green bell pepper (sliced)

1 large red bell pepper (sliced)

1 large yellow bell pepper (sliced)

1 large red onion (sliced)

Directions:

- ➤ Combine the beef, thyme, pepper, garlic, green onion, stock and water in a slow cooker.
- ➤ Leave it all to cook on High for 4 to 5 hours until tender.
- ➤ Remove the beef from the slow cooker and let it cool.
- ➤ Shred the beef with two forks and remove any excess fat.
- ➤ Place the shredded beef back into the slow cooker.
- ➤ Add the sliced peppers and the onion.
- ➤ Cook this on High heat for 40 to 60 minutes until the vegetables are tender.

Nutrition:

Calories - 132

Protein - 14g

Carbohydrates - 9g

Fat - 5g

Cholesterol - 39mg

Sodium - 179mg

Potassium - 390mg

Phosphorus - 141mg

Calcium - 33mg

Fiber - 2g

Sticky Pulled Beef Open Sandwiches

Preparation Time: 15 minutes

Cooking Time: 5 hours

Servings: 5

Ingredients:

½ cup of green onion (sliced)

2 garlic cloves

2 tablespoons of fresh parsley

2 large carrots

7ounce of flat cut beef brisket (whole)

1 tablespoon of smoked paprika

1 teaspoon of dried parsley

1 teaspoon of brown sugar

½ teaspoon of black pepper

2 tablespoons of olive oil

¼ cup of red wine

8 tablespoon of cider vinegar

3 cups of water

5 slices of white bread

1 cup of arugula to garnish

Directions:

- ➢ Finely chop the green onion, garlic and fresh parsley.
- ➢ Grate the carrot.
- ➢ Put the beef in to roast in a slow cooker.
- ➢ Add the chopped onion, garlic and remaining ingredients, leaving the rolls, fresh parsley and arugula to one side.
- ➢ Stir in the slow cooker to combine.
- ➢ Cover and cook on Low for 8 ½ to 10 hours, or on High for 4 to 5 hours until tender. (Hint: Test for tenderness by pressing into the meat with a fork.)
- ➢ Remove the meat from the slow cooker.
- ➢ Shred it apart with two forks.
- ➢ Return the meat to the broth to keep it warm until ready to serve.
- ➢ Lightly toast the bread and top with shredded beef, arugula, fresh parsley and ½ spoon of the broth. Serve.

Nutrition:

Calories – 273 Protein - 15g Carbohydrates - 20g Fat - 11g Cholesterol - 37mg Sodium - 308mg Potassium - 399mg Phosphorus - 159mg Calcium - 113mg Fiber - 3g

Pork Souvlaki

Preparation Time: 20 minutes

Cooking Time: 12 minutes

Servings: 8

Ingredients:

3 tablespoons of olive oil

2 tablespoons of Lemon juice

1 teaspoon of minced garlic

1 tablespoon of chopped fresh oregano

¼ teaspoon of ground black pepper

1 pound Pork leg (cut in 2-inch cubes)

Directions:

➢ In a bowl, stir together the lemon juice, olive oil, garlic, oregano and pepper.

➢ Add the pork cubes and toss to coat.

➢ Place the bowl in the refrigerator, covered for 2 hours to marinate.

➢ Thread the pork chunks onto 8 wooden skewers that have been soaked in water.

➢ Preheat the barbecue to medium-high heat.

➢ Grill the pork skewers for about 12 minutes, turning once, until just cooked through but still juicy.

Nutrition:

Calories - 95

Fat - 4g

Carbs - 0g

Phosphorus - 125mg

Potassium - 230mg

Sodium - 29mg

Protein - 13g

Open-Faced Beef Stir-Up

Preparation Time: 10 minutes

Cooking Time: 10 minutes

Servings: 6

Ingredients:

½ pound of 95% Lean ground beef

½ cup of Chopped sweet onion

½ cup of shredded cabbage

¼ cup of Herb pesto

6 Hamburger buns (bottom halves only)

Directions:

➢ Sauté the beef and onion for 6 minutes or until beef is cooked.
➢ Add the cabbage and sauté for 3 minutes more.
➢ Stir in pesto and heat for 1 minute.
➢ Divide the beef mixture into 6 portions and serve each on the bottom half of a hamburger bun, open-face.

Nutrition:

Calories - 120

Fat - 3g

Phosphorus - 106mg

Potassium - 198mg

Sodium - 134mg

Protein - 11g

Grilled Steak with Cucumber Salsa

Preparation Time: 20 minutes

Cooking Time: 15 minutes

Servings: 4

Ingredients (for the salsa):

1 cup of chopped English cucumber

¼ cup of boiled and diced red bell pepper

Chopped Scallion (both green and white parts)

2 tablespoons of chopped fresh cilantro

Juice from 1 lime

Ingredients (for the steak):

4 (3-ounce) beef tenderloin steaks (room temperature)

Olive oil

Freshly ground black pepper

Directions:

> ➢ To make the salsa, combine the lime juice, cilantro, scallion, bell pepper and cucumber in a bowl. Set aside.
> ➢ To make the steak, preheat a barbecue to medium heat.
> ➢ Rub the steaks all over with oil and season with pepper.
> ➢ Grill the steaks for about 5 minutes per side for medium-rare, or until the desired state.
> ➢ Serve the steaks topped with salsa.

Nutrition:

Calories - 130

Fat - 6g

Carbs - 1g

Phosphorus - 186mg

Potassium - 272mg

Sodium - 39mg

Protein - 19g

Beef Brisket

Preparation Time: 10 minutes

Cooking Time: 3 ½ hours

Servings: 6

Ingredients:

12 ounces of chuck roast (trimmed)

2 cloves of garlic

1 tablespoon of thyme

Rosemary

1 tablespoon of mustard

¼ cup of extra virgin olive oil

1 teaspoon of Black pepper

1 diced Onion

1 cup of peeled, sliced carrots

2 cups of Low salt stock

Directions:

- ➤ Preheat the oven to 300°F.
- ➤ Soak vegetables in warm water.
- ➤ Make a paste by mixing together the thyme, mustard, rosemary and garlic. Then mix in the oil and pepper.
- ➤ Add the beef to the dish.
- ➤ Pour the mixture over the beef into a dish.
- ➤ Place the vegetables onto the bottom of the baking dish around the beef.
- ➤ Cover and roast for 3 hours, or until tender.
- ➤ Uncover the dish and continue to cook for 30 minutes in the oven.
- ➤ Serve.

Nutrition:

Calories - 303

Fat - 25g

Carbs - 7g

Phosphorus - 376mg

Potassium - 246mg

Sodium - 44mg

Protein - 18g

Apricot and Lamb Tagine

Preparation Time: 10 minutes

Cooking Time: 1 to 1 ½ hours

Servings: 2

Ingredients:

1 tablespoon of extra virgin olive oil

2 Lean lamb fillets (cubed)

1 Onion (diced)

4 cups of homemade chicken stock

1 teaspoon of Cumin

1 teaspoon of Turmeric

1 teaspoon of Curry powder

1 teaspoon of dried rosemary

1 teaspoon of chopped parsley

½ cup of canned apricots (juices drained and apricots rinsed)

Directions:

- ➢ Heat the olive oil in a pot.
- ➢ Add lamb to the pot and cook for 5 minutes, or until browned.
- ➢ Remove lamb and set aside.
- ➢ Add the chopped onion to the pot and sauté for 5 minutes, or until it starts to soften.
- ➢ Sprinkle cumin, curry powder and turmeric over the onions, and continue to stir for 4 to 5 minutes.
- ➢ Add the lamb back into the pot with the chicken stock and rosemary.
- ➢ Cover the pot and leave to simmer on a low heat for 1 to 1½ hours or until the lamb is tender and fully cooked through.
- ➢ Add the apricots 15 minutes before the end of the cooking time.
- ➢ Garnish with parsley and serve.

Nutrition:

Calories - 193

Fat - 12g

Carbs - 9g

Phosphorus - 170mg

Potassium - 156mg

Sodium - 105mg

Protein - 20g

Lamb Shoulder with Zucchini and Eggplant

Preparation Time: 10 minutes

Cooking Time: 4 to 5 hours

Servings: 2

Ingredients:

6 ounces of Lean lamb shoulder

2 Zucchinis (cubed)

1 Eggplant (cubed)

1 teaspoon of black pepper

2 tablespoons of extra virgin olive oil

1 tablespoon of Basil

1 tablespoon of Oregano

2 cloves of Garlic (chopped)

Directions:

➢ Preheat the oven to its highest setting.

➢ Soak the vegetables in warm water.

➢ Trim any fat from the lamb shoulder.

➢ Rub the lamb with 1 tablespoon of olive oil, pepper and herbs.

➢ Line a baking tray with the rest of the olive oil, garlic, zucchini and eggplant.

➢ Add the lamb shoulder and cover with foil.

➢ Turn the oven down to 325°F, and add the dish into the oven.

➢ Cook for 4 to 5 hours, remove and rest.

➢ Slice the lamb, and then serve with the vegetables.

Nutrition:

Calories - 478

Fat - 31g

Carbs - 13g

Phosphorus - 197mg

Potassium - 414mg

Sodium - 84mg

Protein - 33g

Beef Chili

Preparation Time: 10 minutes

Cooking Time: 30 minutes

Servings: 2

Ingredients:

1 Onion (diced)

1 red bell pepper (diced)

2 cloves of Garlic (minced)

6 ounces of lean ground beef

1 teaspoon of chili powder

1 teaspoon of Oregano

2 tablespoons of extra virgin olive oil

1 cup of Water

1 cup of Brown rice

1 tablespoon of fresh cilantro (to serve)

Directions:

- ➢ Soak vegetables in warm water.
- ➢ Bring a pan of water to the boil, and add rice for 20 minutes.
- ➢ Meanwhile, add the oil to a pan, and heat on medium-high heat.
- ➢ Add pepper, onions and garlic. Then, sauté for 5 minutes until soft.
- ➢ Remove and set aside.
- ➢ Add beef to the pan and stir until browned.
- ➢ Add vegetables back into the pan, and stir.
- ➢ Now, add chili powder, herbs and water.
- ➢ Cover and turn the heat down a little to simmer for 15 minutes.
- ➢ Meanwhile, drain water from the rice, cover the lid and steam while the chili is cooking.
- ➢ Serve hot with the fresh cilantro sprinkled over the top.

Nutrition:

Calories - 459

Fat - 22g

Carbs - 36g

Phosphorus - 332mg

Potassium - 360mg

Protein - 22g

Turkey Pinwheels

Preparation Time: 10 minutes

Cooking Time: 15 minutes

Servings: 6

Ingredients:

6 toothpicks

8 oz. of spring mix salad greens

1 ten-inch tortilla

2 ounces of thinly sliced deli turkey

9 teaspoon. of whipped cream cheese

1 roasted red bell pepper

Directions:

➢ Cut the red bell pepper into ten strips about a quarter-inch thick.

➢ Spread the whipped cream cheese on the tortilla evenly.

➢ Add the salad greens to create a base layer, then lay the turkey on top of it.

➢ Space out the red bell pepper strips on top of the turkey.

➢ Tuck the end, and begin rolling the tortilla inward.

➢ Use toothpicks to hold the roll into place, and cut it into six pieces.

➢ Serve with the swirl facing upward.

Nutrition:

Calories - 206

Fat - 9g

Carbs - 21g

Protein - 9g

Sodium - 533mg

Potassium - 145mg

Phosphorus - 47mg

Chicken Tacos

Preparation Time: 5 minutes

Cooking Time: 20 minutes

Servings: 4

Ingredients:

8 corn tortillas

1½ teaspoon. of Sodium-free taco seasoning

1 juiced lime

½ cups of cilantro

2 green onions (chopped)

8 oz. of iceberg or romaine lettuce (shredded or chopped)

¼ cup of sour cream

1 pound of boneless and skinless chicken breast

Directions:

➢ Cook chicken by boiling for twenty minutes.

➢ Shred or chop cooked chicken into fine bite-sized pieces.

➢ Mix the seasoning and lime juice with the chicken.

➢ Put chicken mixture and lettuce in tortillas.

➢ Top with green onions, cilantro and sour cream.

Nutrition:

Calories - 260

Fat - 3g

Carbs - 36g

Protein - 23g

Sodium - 922mg

Potassium - 445mg

Phosphorus - 357mg

Tuna Twist

Preparation Time: 10 minutes

Cooking Time: 30 minutes

Servings: 4

Ingredients:

1 can of unsalted or water packaged tuna (drained)

6 teaspoon. of vinegar

½ cup of cooked peas

½ cup celery (chopped)

3 teaspoon. of dried dill weed

12 oz. cooked macaroni

.75 cup of mayonnaise

Directions:

➢ Stir together the macaroni, vinegar and mayonnaise together until blended and smooth.

➢ Stir in remaining ingredients.

➢ Chill before serving.

Nutrition:

Calories - 290

Fat - 10g

Carbs - 32g

Protein - 16g

Sodium - 307mg

Potassium - 175mg

Phosphorus - 111mg

Peanut Butter and Jelly Grilled Sandwich

Preparation Time: 5 minutes

Cooking Time: 5 minutes

Servings: 1

Ingredients:

2 teaspoon. of butter (unsalted)

6 teaspoon. of peanut butter

3 teaspoon. of flavored jelly

2 pieces of bread

Directions:

➢ Spread peanut butter evenly on one bread.
➢ Add the layer of jelly.
➢ Butter the outside of the pieces of bread.
➢ Add the sandwich to a frying pan and toast both sides.

Nutrition:

Calories - 300

Fat - 7g

Carbs - 49g

Protein - 8g

Sodium - 460mg

Potassium - 222mg

Phosphorus - 80mg

Grilled Onion and Pepper Jack Grilled Cheese Sandwich

Preparation Time: 5 minutes

Cooking Time: 5 minutes

Servings: 2

Ingredients:

1 teaspoon. of olive oil

6 teaspoon. of whipped cream cheese

½ of a medium onion

2 ounces of pepper jack cheese

4 slices of rye bread

2 teaspoon. of unsalted butter

Directions:

➤ Set out the butter so that it becomes soft.

➤ Slice up the onion into thin slices.

➤ Sauté onion slices and continue to stir until cooked.

➤ Remove and put it to the side.

➤ Spread one tablespoon of whipped cream cheese on two of the slices of bread.

➤ Then, add grilled onions and cheese to each slice, and top using the other two bread slices.

➤ Spread the softened butter on the outside of the slices of bread.

➤ Use the skillet to toast the sandwiches until lightly brown and the cheese is melted.

Nutrition:

Calories - 350

Fat - 18g

Carbs - 34g

Protein - 13g

Sodium - 589mg

Potassium - 184mg

Phosphorus - 226mg

Carrot & Ginger Chicken Noodles

Preparation Time: 5 minutes

Cooking Time: 10 minutes

Servings: 4

Ingredients:

1 sliced green onion

2 teaspoon. of grated fresh ginger

4 oz. skinless sliced chicken breasts

1 lime

1 minced garlic clove

1 cup of cooked rice noodles

1 teaspoon. coconut oil

1 peeled and grated carrot

Directions:

➢ Heat a large pan over medium to high heat.
➢ Add the coconut oil to a pan, and once melted, add the sliced chicken and brown for 4 to 5 minutes.
➢ Now, add the ginger and garlic and sauté for 4 to 5 minutes.
➢ Add green onion, carrot and lime juice to the wok.
➢ Put the cooked noodles into the pan, and toss until hot through.
➢ Serve hot and enjoy.

Nutrition:

Calories - 187

Protein - 11 g

Carbs - 25 g

Fat - 5 g

Sodium - 39 mg

Potassium - 91 mg

Phosphorus - 178 mg

Ginger & Bean Sprout Steak Stir-Fry

Preparation Time: 4 minutes

Cooking Time: 10 minutes

Servings: 2

Ingredients:

2 teaspoon. of grated fresh ginger

1 teaspoon. of coconut oil

1 teaspoon. of nutmeg

1 finely sliced green onion

¼ cup of bean sprouts

5 oz. of sliced lean organic beef steak

1 minced garlic clove

Directions:

➢ Add the strip beef into a dry, hot pan and cook for 4-5 minutes on each side or until they're cooked to your liking; then, set aside.

➢ Add the oil to a clean pan and sauté the bean sprouts and onions with ginger, garlic and nutmeg for 1 minute.

➢ Serve the beef strips on a bed of vegetables and enjoy.

Nutrition:

Calories - 227

Protein - 13 g

Carbs - 13 g

Fat - 23 g

Sodium - 50 mg

Potassium - 258 mg

Phosphorus - 170 mg

Lemon & Herb Chicken Wraps

Preparation Time: 5 minutes

Cooking Time: 30 minutes

Servings: 4

Ingredients:

4 oz. skinless and sliced chicken breasts

½ sliced red bell pepper

1 lemon

4 large iceberg lettuce leaves

1 tablespoon. of olive oil

2 tablespoons of finely chopped fresh cilantro

¼ teaspoon. of black pepper

Directions:

- ➤ Preheat the oven to 375°F.
- ➤ Mix the oil, juice of ½ lemon, cilantro and black pepper.
- ➤ Marinate the chicken in the oil marinade, cover, and leave in the fridge for as long as possible.
- ➤ Wrap the chicken in parchment paper, drizzling over the remaining marinade.
- ➤ Place in the oven in an oven dish for 25-30 minutes, or until chicken is thoroughly cooked through, and white inside.
- ➤ Divide the sliced bell pepper and layer onto each lettuce leaf.
- ➤ Divide the chicken onto each lettuce leaf, and squeeze over the remaining lemon juice to taste.

- ➤ Wrap and enjoy.

Nutrition:

Calories - 364

Protein - 35g

Carbs - 32g

Fat - 10g

Sodium - 398mg

Potassium - 413mg

Phosphorus - 264mg

Chinese Beef Wraps

Preparation Time: 10 minutes

Cooking Time: 30 minutes

Servings: 2

Ingredients:

2 iceberg lettuce leaves

½ diced cucumber

1 teaspoon. of canola oil

5 oz. of lean ground beef

1 teaspoon. of ground ginger

1 tablespoon. chili flakes

1 minced garlic clove

1 tablespoon. of rice wine vinegar

Directions:

➢ Mix the ground meat with the garlic, rice wine vinegar, chili flakes and ginger in a bowl.

➢ Get a skillet and heat over medium flame.

➢ Add the beef to the pan, and cook for 20 to 25 minutes, or until cooked through.

➢ Serve beef mixture with diced cucumber in each lettuce wrap and fold.

Nutrition:

Calories - 205

Fat - 12g

Carbs - 16g

Protein - 8.7g

Sodium - 347mg

Phosphorus - 101mg

Potassium - 408mg

CHAPTER 11:

Snacks Recipes

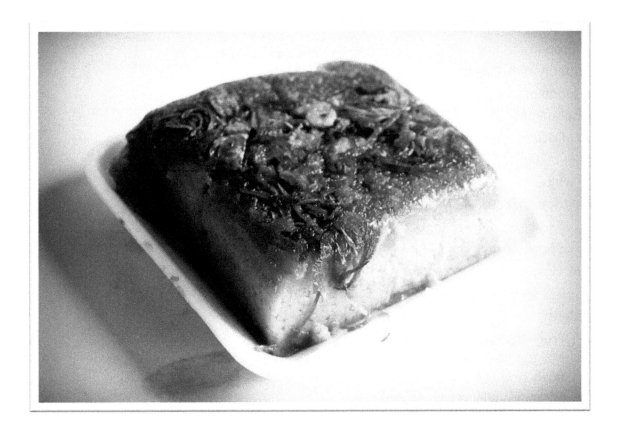

Spicy Corn Bread

Preparation Time: 10 minutes

Cooking Time: 30 minutes

Servings: 8

Ingredients:

1 cup of all-purpose white flour

1 cup of plain cornmeal

1 tablespoon of sugar

2 teaspoons of baking powder

1 teaspoon of chili powder

¼ teaspoon of black pepper

1 cup of rice milk (unenriched)

1 egg

1 egg white

2 tablespoons of canola oil

½ cup of scallions (finely chopped)

¼ cup of finely grated carrots

1 garlic clove (minced)

Directions:

➢ Preheat your oven to 400ºF.
➢ Mix the flour with baking powder, sugar, cornmeal, pepper and chili powder in a mixing bowl.
➢ Stir in oil, milk, egg white and egg.
➢ Mix well until it is smooth, then stir in carrots, garlic and scallions.
➢ Stir well, then spread the batter in an 8-inch baking pan greased with cooking spray.
➢ Bake for 30 minutes until golden brown.
➢ Slice and serve fresh.

Nutrition:

Calories – 188 Protein - 5 g

Carbohydrates - 31 g Fat - 5 g

Cholesterol - 26 mg Sodium - 155 mg

Potassium - 100 mg

Phosphorus - 81 mg

Calcium - 84 mg Fiber - 2 g

Sweet and Spicy Tortilla Chips

Preparation Time: 10 minutes

Cooking Time: 8 minutes

Servings: 6

Ingredients:

¼ cup of butter

1 teaspoon of brown sugar

½ teaspoon of ground chili powder

½ teaspoon of garlic powder

½ teaspoon of ground cumin

¼ teaspoon of ground cayenne pepper

6 flour tortillas (6" size)

Directions:

- ➢ Preheat oven to 425°F.
- ➢ Grease a baking sheet with cooking spray.
- ➢ Add all spices, brown sugar and melted butter to a small bowl.
- ➢ Mix well, and set this mixture aside.
- ➢ Slice the tortillas into 8 wedges, and brush them with the sugar mixture.
- ➢ Spread them on the baking sheet, and bake them for 8 minutes.
- ➢ Serve fresh.

Nutrition:

Calories - 115

Protein - 2 g

Carbohydrates - 11 g

Fat - 7 g

Cholesterol - 15 mg

Sodium - 156 mg

Potassium - 42 mg

Phosphorus - 44 mg

Calcium - 31 mg

Fiber - 0.6 g

Addictive Pretzels

Preparation Time: 10 minutes
Cooking Time: 1 hour
Servings: 6

Ingredients:
32-ounce bag unsalted pretzels
1 cup of canola oil
2 tablespoons of seasoning mix
3 teaspoons of garlic powder
3 teaspoons of dried dill weed

Directions:
- ➢ Preheat oven to 175ºF.
- ➢ Place the pretzels on a cooking sheet, and break them into pieces.
- ➢ Mix garlic powder and dill in a bowl, and reserve half of the mixture.
- ➢ Mix the remaining half with seasoning mix and ¾ cup of canola oil.
- ➢ Pour this oil over the pretzels, and brush them liberally.
- ➢ Bake the pieces for 1 hour, then flip them to bake for another 15 minutes.
- ➢ Allow them to cool, then sprinkle the remaining dill mixture, and drizzle more oil on top.
- ➢ Serve fresh and warm.

Nutrition:
Calories - 184
Protein - 2 g
Carbohydrates - 22 g
Fat - 8 g
Cholesterol - 0 mg
Sodium - 60 mg
Potassium - 43 mg
Phosphorus - 28 mg
Calcium - 2 mg
Fiber - 1.0 g

Cream Dipped Cucumbers

Preparation Time: 5 minutes

Cooking Time: 0 minutes

Servings: 4

Ingredients:

½ cup of sour cream

3 tablespoons of white vinegar

1 teaspoon of stevia

Pepper to taste

4 cucumbers (peeled and sliced)

1 small sweet onion, cut in rings

Directions:

➢ Use a medium-sized serving bowl.
➢ Add in the cucumber, onion and all the other ingredients.
➢ Mix them well, and refrigerate for 2 hours.
➢ Toss again, serve and enjoy.

Nutrition:

Calories - 127

Total Fat - 6.4g

Saturated Fat - 3.9g

Cholesterol - 13mg

Sodium - 23mg

Carbohydrate - 9.2g

Dietary Fiber - 1.9g

Sugars - 4.2g

Protein - 3.1g

Calcium - 86mg

Phosphorous - 172mg

Potassium - 518mg

Barbecue Cups

Preparation Time: 5 minutes

Cooking Time: 20 minutes

Servings: 10

Ingredients:

¾ lb. of lean ground turkey

½ cup of spicy barbecue sauce

2 teaspoons of onion flakes

A dash of garlic powder

1 (10-oz.) package of low-fat biscuits

Directions:

➢ Grease a suitable pan with cooking spray, and place it over moderate heat.

➢ Add the ground turkey, and sauté it until golden brown.

➢ Flatten the biscuits, and place them in a muffin tray.

➢ Press each biscuit in its muffin cup, and divide the turkey in them.

➢ Top the turkey with barbecue sauce, garlic powder and onion flakes.

➢ Bake for 12 minutes at 400°F in a preheated oven.

➢ Serve.

Nutrition:

Calories - 143

Total Fat - 6.3g

Saturated Fat - 1.8g

Cholesterol - 25mg

Sodium - 329mg

Carbohydrate - 13.1g

Dietary Fiber - 0.2g

Sugars - 2.7g

Protein - 8.6g

Calcium - 21mg

Phosphorous - 367mg

Potassium - 164mg

Spiced Pretzels

Preparation Time: 5 minutes

Cooking Time: 1 hour 15 minutes

Servings: 10

Ingredients:

1 teaspoon of ground cayenne pepper

1 teaspoon of lemon pepper

1 ½ teaspoons of garlic powder

1 oz. of dry ranch-style dressing

¾ cup of vegetable oil

15 oz. packages of mini pretzels

Directions:

➢ Switch the oven to 175°F to preheat.

➢ Spread the pretzels on a cooking sheet and break them into pieces.

➢ Whisk the oil with the garlic powder, lemon pepper, ground cayenne pepper and ranch dressing in a bowl.

➢ Pour this oil dressing over the pretzels, and toss well to coat.

➢ Bake the pretzels for approximately 1 hour, then flip them to bake for another 15 minutes.

➢ Serve fresh and warm.

Nutrition:

Calories - 311

Total Fat - 18.6g

Saturated Fat - 3.2g

Cholesterol - 0mg

Sodium - 270mg

Carbohydrate - 33.2g

Dietary Fiber - 1.6g

Sugars - 0g

Protein - 3g

Calcium - 1mg

Phosphorous - 371mg

Potassium - 6mg

Cauliflower with Mustard Sauce

Preparation Time: 5 minutes

Cooking Time: 10 minutes

Servings: 4

Ingredients:

1 head of cauliflower, separated into florets

½ cup of mayonnaise

¼ cup of Dijon mustard

1 cup of sharp cheddar cheese (shredded)

Directions:

- ➢ Whisk the mayonnaise with the mustard and cheese in a bowl.
- ➢ Add the cauliflower florets in boiling water in a pot, and cook until they are tender.
- ➢ Drain the cauliflower, then toss its florets with the mayo mixture.
- ➢ Spread the cauliflower mixture in a baking pan.
- ➢ Broil it for 5 minutes until the cheese is melted.
- ➢ Serve fresh.

Nutrition:

Calories - 255

Total Fat - 19.9g

Saturated Fat - 7.5g

Cholesterol - 37mg

Sodium - 582mg

Carbohydrate - 11.7g

Dietary Fiber - 2.2g

Sugars - 3.8g

Protein - 9.3g

Calcium - 231mg

Phosphorous - 97mg

Potassium - 253mg

Pineapple Cabbage Coleslaw

Preparation Time: 5 minutes

Cooking Time: 0 minutes

Servings: 12

Ingredients:

12 oz. (bag) of broccoli coleslaw

12 oz. of finely shredded Napa cabbage

20 oz. (can) of drained unsweetened pineapple

½ cup of green onions (sliced)

1 cup of mayonnaise

1 tablespoon of seasoned rice vinegar

1 teaspoon of coarse ground black pepper

Directions:

➢ Toss the cabbage with the broccoli and all the other ingredients in a salad bowl.

➢ Refrigerate this coleslaw for at least 1 hour.

➢ Serve.

Nutrition:

Calories - 186

Total Fat - 12.7g

Saturated Fat - 2g

Cholesterol - 5mg

Sodium - 224mg

Carbohydrate - 18g

Dietary Fiber - 2.1g

Sugars - 10.4g

Protein - 2g

Calcium - 42mg

Phosphorous - 106mg

Potassium - 139mg

Seafood Croquettes

Preparation Time: 10 minutes

Cooking Time: 20 minutes

Servings: 8

Ingredients:

14.75 oz. of packed salmon

2 egg whites

¼ cup of chopped onion

½ teaspoon of black pepper

½ cup of plain breadcrumbs

2 tablespoons of lemon juice

½ teaspoon of ground mustard

¼ cup of regular mayonnaise

Directions:

➢ Drain the packed salmon and transfer it to a bowl.
➢ Stir in all the other ingredients except the oil and mix well.
➢ Make 8 patties out of this mixture and keep them aside.
➢ Add the oil to a pan, and place it over medium-high heat.
➢ Add 4 patties at a time and sear them for 3 minutes per side.
➢ Cook the remaining four in the same manner until golden brown.
➢ Serve.

Nutrition:

Calories - 282

Total Fat - 12g

Saturated Fat - 2.6g

Cholesterol - 66mg

Sodium - 202mg

Carbohydrate - 7.4g

Dietary Fiber - 0.4g

Sugars - 1.3g

Protein - 12.6g

Calcium - 88mg

Phosphorous - 137mg

Potassium - 253mg

Sweet Rice Salad

Preparation Time: 5 minutes

Cooking Time: 0 minutes

Servings: 6

Ingredients:

3 tablespoons of apricot jam

1 tablespoon of water

1 tablespoon of lemon juice

7 tablespoons of mayonnaise

6 oz. of long-grain rice, cooked & rinsed

1 oz. of finely chopped onion

2 apples (chopped)

8 cherry tomatoes

Directions:

➢ Mix the rice with apples, tomatoes and onion in a salad bowl.

➢ Whisk the apricot jam and the rest of the dressing ingredients in a small bowl.

➢ Pour this dressing into the rice salad and mix well.

➢ Serve.

Nutrition:

Calories - 265

Total Fat - 6.4g

Saturated Fat - 1g

Cholesterol - 4mg

Sodium - 137mg

Carbohydrate - 49.2g

Dietary Fiber - 4.3g

Sugars - 17.8g

Protein - 4g

Calcium - 30mg

Phosphorous - 258mg

Potassium - 520mg

Shrimp Spread with Crackers

Preparation Time: 10 minutes

Cooking Time: 0 minutes

Servings: 6

Ingredients:

¼ cup of light cream cheese

2 ½ ounce of cooked, shelled shrimp (minced)

1 tablespoon of ketchup (no salt added)

¼ teaspoon of hot sauce

1 teaspoon of Worcestershire sauce

½ teaspoon of herb seasoning blend

24 matzo cracker miniatures

1 tablespoon of parsley

Directions:

- ➤ Start by tossing the minced shrimp with cream cheese in a bowl.
- ➤ Stir in Worcestershire sauce, hot sauce, herb seasoning and ketchup.
- ➤ Mix well, and garnish with minced parsley.
- ➤ Serve the spread with the crackers.

Nutrition:

Calories - 57

Protein - 3 g

Carbohydrates - 7 g

Fat - 1 g

Cholesterol - 21 mg

Sodium - 69 mg

Potassium - 54 mg

Phosphorus - 30 mg

Calcium - 15 mg

Fiber - 0.2 g

Buffalo Chicken Dip

Preparation Time: 10 minutes

Cooking Time: 3 hours

Servings: 4

Ingredients:

4-ounce of cream cheese

½ cup of bottled roasted red peppers

1 cup of low-fat sour cream

4 teaspoons of hot pepper sauce

2 cups of cooked, shredded chicken

Directions:

➢ Blend half cup of drained red peppers in a food processor until smooth.

➢ Now, thoroughly mix cream cheese and sour cream with the pureed peppers in a bowl.

➢ Stir in shredded chicken and hot sauce, then transfer the mixture to a slow cooker.

➢ Cook for 3 hours on low heat.

➢ Serve warm with celery, carrots, cauliflower and cucumber.

Nutrition:

Calories - 73

Protein - 5 g

Carbohydrates - 2 g

Fat - 5 g

Cholesterol - 25 mg

Sodium - 66 mg

Potassium - 81 mg

Phosphorus - 47 mg

Calcium - 31 mg

Fiber - 0 g

Chicken Pepper Bacon Wraps

Preparation Time: 10 minutes

Cooking Time: 15 minutes

Servings: 4

Ingredients:

1 medium onion (chopped)

12 strips of bacon (halved)

12 fresh jalapenos peppers

12 fresh banana peppers

2 pounds of boneless, skinless chicken breast

Directions:

- ➤ Grease a grill rack with cooking spray, and preheat the grill on low heat.
- ➤ Slice the peppers in half lengthwise, then remove their seeds.
- ➤ Dice the chicken into small pieces, and divide them into each pepper.
- ➤ Now spread the chopped onion over the chicken in the peppers.
- ➤ Wrap the bacon strips around the stuffed peppers.
- ➤ Place these wrapped peppers in the grill, and cook them for 15 minutes.
- ➤ Serve fresh and warm.

Nutrition:

Calories - 71

Protein - 10 g

Carbohydrates - 1 g

Fat - 3 g

Cholesterol - 26 mg

Sodium - 96 mg

Potassium - 147 mg

Phosphorus - 84 mg

Calcium - 9 mg

Fiber - 0.8 g

Garlic Oyster Crackers

Preparation Time: 10 minutes

Cooking Time: 45 minutes

Servings: 4

Ingredients:

½ cup of butter-flavored popcorn oil

1 tablespoon of garlic powder

7 cups of oyster crackers

2 teaspoons of dried dill weed

Directions:

➢ Preheat oven to 250°F.

➢ Mix garlic powder with oil in a large bowl.

➢ Toss in crackers and mix well to coat evenly.

➢ Sprinkle the dill weed over the crackers, and toss well again.

➢ Spread the crackers on the baking sheet, and bake them for 45 minutes.

➢ Toss them every 15 minutes.

➢ Serve fresh.

Nutrition:

Calories - 118

Protein - 2 g

Carbohydrates - 12 g

Fat - 7 g

Cholesterol - 0 mg

Sodium - 166 mg

Potassium - 21 mg

Phosphorus - 15 mg

Calcium - 4 mg

Fiber - 3 g

CHAPTER 12:

Dinner Recipes

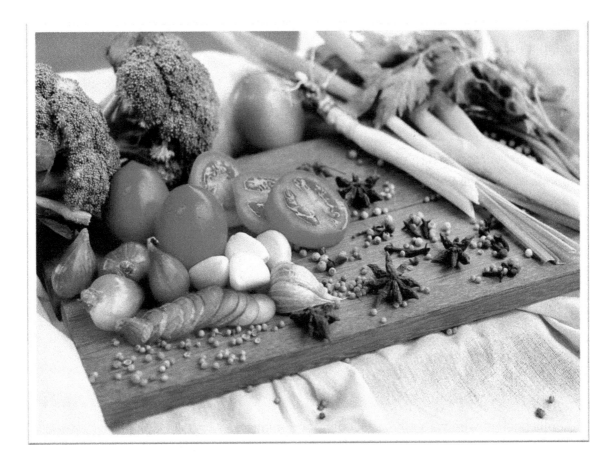

Eggplant Seafood Casserole

Preparation Time: 10 minutes

Cooking Time: 20 minutes

Servings: 4

Ingredients:

2 medium eggplants (diced)

1 medium onion (diced)

1 bell pepper (diced)

½ cup of chopped celery

2 garlic cloves (minced)

¼ cup of olive oil

¼ cup of lemon juice

1 tablespoon of Worcestershire sauce

¼ teaspoons of salt-free Creole seasoning

½ teaspoon of hot pepper sauce

⅓ cup of uncooked rice

¼ cup of Parmesan cheese

1 dash of cayenne pepper

3 eggs - 1 lb. of lump crab meat

½ lb. of boiled shrimp

½ cup of breadcrumbs

2 tablespoons of unsalted butter (melted)

Directions:

➢ Boil eggplant with water in a saucepan for 5 minutes.

➢ Drain the eggplant and keep it aside. Now, sauté the onion with celery, bell pepper, garlic and oil in the Instant Pot on Sauté mode.

➢ Transfer these veggies to the eggplant, along with all other ingredients except the breadcrumbs.

➢ Mix well, then spread this mixture into a casserole dish suitable to fit in the Instant Pot.

➢ Pour 1½ cup of water into the Instant pot, and place a trivet over it.

➢ Set the casserole dish over the trivet. Spread the crumbs over the casserole.

➢ Seal the lid, and cook for 15 minutes on Manual mode at High pressure.

➢ Remove the pot's lid when done, and serve warm.

Nutrition:

Calories – 216 Fats - 12 g Carbs - 14 g Fiber - 2.3 g Protein - 13 g

Sodium - 482mg Potassium - 690mg Phosphorus - 182mg

Halibut with Lemon Caper Sauce

Preparation Time: 10 minutes
Cooking Time: 10 minutes
Servings: 4

Ingredients:
4 tablespoons of lemon juice
1 tablespoon of olive oil
20 oz. of raw halibut steaks
2 tablespoons of unsalted butter
2 teaspoons of almond flour
½ cup of low-sodium chicken broth
¼ cup of white wine
1 teaspoon of capers
¼ teaspoon of white pepper

Directions:
- ➢ Season the halibut steaks with 2 tablespoons lemon juice and olive oil in a bowl.
- ➢ Now, melt butter in the instant pot on Sauté mode.
- ➢ Stir in the remaining ingredients and whisk well.
- ➢ Place a steamer basket over the sauce mixture, and add halibut to the basket.
- ➢ Seal the lid and cook for 5 minutes on Manual mode at High pressure.
- ➢ Once done, release the pressure completely, then remove the pot's lid.
- ➢ Remove the fish and the basket.
- ➢ Add the fish to the sauce, and mix well gently.
- ➢ Serve warm.

Nutrition:
Calories - 260
Fats - 10g
Carbs - 5g
Protein - 36g
Sodium - 118 mg
Potassium - 573mg
Phosphorus - 306mg

Jambalaya

Preparation Time: 10 minutes

Cooking Time: 25 minutes

Servings: 4

Ingredients:

2 cups of onion

1 cup of bell pepper

2 garlic cloves

2 cups of converted white rice (uncooked)

½ teaspoon of black pepper

8 oz. of canned low-sodium tomato sauce

2 cups of low-sodium beef broth

2 lbs. of raw shrimp

½ cup of margarine

Directions:

- ➢ Toss all the ingredients except margarine in a baking dish.
- ➢ Place the margarine slice on top of the mixture.
- ➢ Cover the dish with an aluminum foil.
- ➢ Pour 1½ cups over into the instant pot, and set the trivet over it.
- ➢ Place the prepared baking dish over the trivet.
- ➢ Press manual mode at high pressure and seal the lid.
- ➢ Cook for 25 minutes.
- ➢ Once done, release the pressure, and gently remove the pot's lid.
- ➢ Serve warm.

Nutrition:

Calories - 207

Fats - 4g

Carbs - 30g

Fiber - 1.5g

Protein - 12g

Sodium - 462mg

Potassium - 304mg

Phosphorus - 107mg

Raw Vegetables; Chopped Salad

Preparation Time: 15 minutes

Cooking Time: 0 minute

Servings: 4

Ingredients:

Chopped raw veggie salad

1 orange pepper (minced) (about 1 cup)

1 yellow pepper (small cut) (about 1 cup)

5-8 radishes (halve and cut into thin slices) (about ¾ cup)

Small head of broccoli (minced) (about 2 cups)

1 seedless cucumber (small cut) (about 2 cups)

1 cup of halved red seedless grapes

2 to 3 tablespoons of chopped fresh dill

¼ cup of chopped fresh parsley

¼ cup of raw peeled sunflower seeds

⅛ cup raw hemp hearts (peeled hemp seeds)

Oil-free dressing

Garlic clove (chopped)

Tablespoons of red wine vinegar

1 tablespoon of apple cider vinegar

Juice of 1 lemon - 1 tablespoon of Dijonsenf

1 tablespoon of pure maple syrup

½ teaspoon of salt (or to taste)

⅛ teaspoon of pepper (or to taste)

Directions:

➢ Whisk the ingredients - Chopped raw veggie salad, 1 orange pepper, yellow pepper, radishes, small head of broccoli, seedless cucumber, halved red seedless grapes, chopped fresh dill, chopped fresh parsley, raw peeled sunflower seeds, raw hemp hearts, garlic clove, red wine vinegar, apple cider vinegar, lemon, Dijonsenf, pure maple syrup, salt, pepper. For dressing in a small bowl and set aside.

➢ Mix all the salad ingredients in a large bowl. Pour the dressing over and wrap well.

➢ Cover and then refrigerate it for an hour or two (toss the salad once or twice during this time to coat evenly). Enjoy!

Nutrition:

Calories - 111 Total Fat - 2g Saturated Fat - 1g Cholesterol - 10mg

Sodium - 58mg Carbohydrates - 19g Sugar - 18 g Calcium - 15%

Turkey Sausages

Preparation Time: 10 minutes

Cooking Time: 10 minutes

Servings: 2

Ingredients:

¼ teaspoon of salt

⅛ teaspoon of garlic powder

⅛ teaspoon of onion powder

1 teaspoon of fennel seed

1 pound of 7% fat ground turkey

Directions:

- ➢ Press the fennel seed.
- ➢ In a small cup put together turkey with fennel seed, garlic, onion powder and salt.
- ➢ Cover the bowl and refrigerate overnight.
- ➢ Prepare the turkey with seasoning into different portions with a circle form, and press them into patties ready to be cooked.
- ➢ Cook at a medium heat until browned.
- ➢ Cook it for 1 to 2 minutes per side, and serve them hot. Enjoy!

Nutrition:

Calories - 55

Protein - 7 g

Sodium - 70 mg

Potassium - 105 mg

Phosphorus - 75 mg

Rosemary Chicken

Preparation Time: 10 minutes

Cooking Time: 10 minutes

Servings: 2

Ingredients:

2 zucchinis

1 carrot

1 teaspoon of dried rosemary

4 chicken breasts

½ bell pepper

½ red onion

8 garlic cloves

Olive oil

¼ tablespoon of ground pepper

Directions:

➢ Prepare the oven, and preheat it at 375°F (or 200°C).
➢ Slice both zucchini and carrots. Then, add bell pepper, onion and garlic.
➢ Put everything in a 13" x 9" pan, and add oil.
➢ Spread the pepper over everything, and roast for about 10 minutes.
➢ Meanwhile, lift up the chicken skin, and spread black pepper and rosemary on the flesh.
➢ Remove the vegetable pan from the oven and add the chicken, returning the pan to the oven for about 30 more minutes.
➢ Serve and enjoy!

Nutrition:

Calories - 215

Protein - 28 g

Sodium - 105 mg

Potassium - 580 mg

Phosphorus - 250 mg

Smoky Turkey Chili

Preparation Time: 5 minutes

Cooking Time: 45 minutes

Servings: 8

Ingredients:

12ounce lean ground turkey

½ red onion (chopped)

2 cloves of garlic (crushed and chopped)

½ teaspoon of smoked paprika

½ teaspoon of chili powder

½ teaspoon of dried thyme

¼ cup of low-sodium beef stock

½ cup of water

1 ½ cups of baby spinach leaves, washed

3 wheat tortillas

Directions:

- ➢ Brown the ground beef in a dry skillet over a medium-high heat.
- ➢ Add in the red onion and garlic.
- ➢ Sauté the onion until it goes clear.
- ➢ Transfer the contents of the skillet to the slow cooker.
- ➢ Add the remaining ingredients and simmer on Low for 30 to 45 minutes.
- ➢ Stir through the spinach for the last few minutes to wilt.
- ➢ Slice tortillas and gently toast under the broiler until slightly crispy.
- ➢ Serve on top of the turkey chili.

Nutrition:

Calories - 93.5

Protein - 8g

Carbohydrates - 3g

Fat - 5.5g

Cholesterol - 30.5mg

Sodium - 84.5mg

Potassium - 142.5mg

Phosphorus - 92.5mg

Calcium - 29mg

Fiber - 0.5g

Mediterranean Veggie Pita Sandwich

Preparation Time: 4hours, 30mins

Cooking Time: 30 minutes

Servings: 2

Ingredients:

¼ cup of chopped carrots

A handful of baby spinach

¼ cup of chickpeas

1 teaspoon of crumbled feta cheese

2 teaspoons of fine chopped sun-dried tomatoes

2 teaspoons of chopped kalamata olives

Season with salt and pepper

Directions:

- ➢ The chopped carrots, baby spinach, chickpeas, crumbled feta cheese, chopped sun-dried tomatoes, chopped kalamata olives, salt and pepper.
- ➢ Spread the bath in every pita pant.
- ➢ Sort the rest of the ingredients between the boxes.
- ➢ Eat immediately, or pack in a container for lunch.
- ➢ Cool the device if you prepare it for more than 4 hours before eating.

Nutrition:

Calories - 287.6

Sodium - 716.0 mg

Potassium - 263.6 mg

Total Carbohydrate - 45.7 g

Dietary Fiber - 6.8 g

Cauliflower and Asparagus Tortilla

Preparation Time: 10 minutes

Cooking Time: 30 minutes

Servings: 4

Ingredients:

2 cups of Asparagus

2 cups of Cauliflower

2 teaspoons of Olive oil

1½ cups of Onion

1 clove of Garlic

1 cup of liquid egg substitute (low-cholesterol)

2 tablespoons of fresh parsley (finely chopped)

¼ teaspoon of Salt

½ teaspoon of freshly ground Pepper

¼ teaspoon of dried thyme leaves (crushed)

¼ teaspoon of ground nutmeg

Directions:

➢ Start by chopping the asparagus and cauliflower into 1-inch pieces. Take the onion and chop it finely. Also, mince the garlic clove.

➢ Take a microwave-safe bowl, and place the chopped cauliflower and asparagus pieces into it. Add in 1 tablespoon of water and cover the dish.

➢ After that, drain any excess water and set aside.

➢ Microwave them for about 4-5 minutes. Make sure the veggies are slightly tender.

➢ Place a saucepan over a high flame and pour the oil into it. Once heated, toss in the finely chopped onions.

➢ Sauté the onions for about 6 to 7 minutes. Add in the minced garlic, and sauté for 1 more minute.

➢ Toss in the cauliflower, asparagus, egg substitute, salt, thyme, parsley and nutmeg. Arrange them well over the egg substitute base.

➢ Cover the saucepan, and cook for about 15 minutes in low heat.

➢ Use a butter knife to loosen the edges of the prepared tortilla.

➢ Take a microwave-safe serving platter and heat it for about 30 to 40 seconds.

➢ Invert the tortilla onto the heated serving platter. Serve hot!

Nutrition:

Protein - 9 g Fat - 3 g Carbohydrates - 9 g

Sodium - 248 mg Cholesterol - 0 mg

Potassium - 472 mg Calcium - 68 mg Phosphorus - 97 mg Fiber - 3.88 g

Avocado-Orange Grilled Chicken

Preparation Time: 20 minutes

Cooking Time: 60 minutes

Servings: 4

Ingredients:

¼ cup of fresh lime juice

¼ cup of minced red onion

1 avocado

1 cup of low fat yogurt

1 small red onion, sliced thinly

1 tablespoon of honey

2 oranges, peeled and sectioned

2 tablespoons of chopped cilantro

4 pieces of 4-6ounce boneless, skinless chicken breasts

Pepper and salt to taste

Directions:

➢ Mix honey, cilantro, minced red onion and yogurt in a large bowl.
➢ Submerge chicken into mixture, and marinate for at least 30 minutes.
➢ Grease grate and preheat grill to medium high fire.
➢ Remove chicken from marinade and season with pepper and salt.
➢ Grill for 6 minutes per side, or until chicken is cooked and juices run clear.
➢ Meanwhile, peel avocado and discard seed. Then, chop and place in bowl.
➢ Quickly add lime juice and toss avocado to coat well with juice.
➢ Add cilantro, thinly sliced onions and oranges into bowl of avocado, and mix well.
➢ Serve grilled chicken and avocado dressing on the side.

Nutrition:

Calories - 209

Carbs - 26g

Protein - 8g

Fats - 10g

Phosphorus - 157mg

 Potassium - 548mg

Sodium - 125mg

Chicken & Cauliflower Rice Casserole

Preparation Time: 15 minutes

Cooking Time: 1 hour, 15 minutes

Servings: 8 to 10

Ingredients:

2 tablespoons of coconut oil, divided

3-pound bone-in chicken thighs and drumsticks

Salt and freshly ground black pepper, to taste

3 carrots, peeled and sliced

1 onion (chopped finely)

2 garlic cloves (chopped finely)

2 tablespoons of fresh cinnamon, (chopped finely)

2 teaspoons of ground cumin

1 teaspoon of ground coriander

12 teaspoons of ground cinnamon

½ teaspoon of ground turmeric

1 teaspoon of paprika - ¼ teaspoon of red pepper cayenne

1 (28-ounce) can of diced tomatoes with liquid

1 red bell pepper, seeded and cut into thin strips

½ cup of fresh parsley leaves (minced)

Salt, to taste - 1 head cauliflower, grated to some rice like consistency

1 lemon, sliced thinly

Directions:

➢ Preheat the oven to 375°F. In a large pan, melt 1 tablespoon of coconut oil at high heat.

➢ Add chicken pieces and cook for about 3 to 5 minutes per side, or till golden brown.

➢ Transfer the chicken in a plate.

➢ In a similar pan, sauté the carrot, onion, garlic and ginger for about 4 to 5 minutes on medium heat. Stir in spices and remaining coconut oil.

➢ Add chicken, tomatoes, bell pepper, parsley and salt. Then, simmer for approximately 3 to 5 minutes.

➢ In the bottom of a 13x9-inch rectangular baking dish, spread the cauliflower rice evenly.

➢ Place chicken mixture over cauliflower rice evenly, and top with lemon slices.

➢ With a foil paper, cover the baking dish, and bake for approximately 35 minutes.

➢ Uncover the baking dish and bake for approximately 25 minutes.

Nutrition:

Calories – 412 Fat - 12g Carbohydrates - 23g

Fiber - 7g Protein - 34g Phosphorus - 297 mg Potassium - 811 mg Sodium - 711 mg

Grilled Squash

Preparation Time: 10 minutes

Cooking Time: 6 minutes

Servings: 8

Ingredients:

4 zucchinis, rinsed, drained and sliced

4 crookneck squash, rinsed, drained and sliced

Cooking spray

¼ teaspoon of garlic powder

¼ teaspoon of black pepper

Directions:

> ➢ Arrange squash on a baking sheet.
> ➢ Spray with oil.
> ➢ Season with garlic powder and pepper.
> ➢ Grill for 3 minutes per side, or until tender but not too soft.

Nutrition:

Calories - 17

Protein - 1 g

Carbohydrates - 3 g

Fat - 0 g

Cholesterol - 0 mg

Sodium - 6 mg

Potassium - 262 mg

Phosphorus - 39 mg

Calcium - 16 mg

 Fiber - 1.1 g

Thai Tofu Broth

Preparation Time: 5 minutes
Cooking Time: 15 minutes
Servings: 4

Ingredients:
1 cup of rice noodles
½ sliced onion
6 ounce drained, pressed and cubed tofu
¼ cup of sliced scallions
½ cup of water
½ cup of canned water chestnuts
½ cup of rice milk
1 tablespoon of lime juice
1 tablespoon of coconut oil
½ finely sliced chili
1 cup of snow peas

Directions:
- Heat the oil in a wok on a high heat. Then, sauté the tofu until brown on each side.
- Add the onion and sauté for 2 to 3 minutes.
- Add the rice milk and water to the wok until bubbling.
- Lower to medium heat, and add the noodles, chili and water chestnuts.
- Allow to simmer for 10 to15 minutes. Then, add sugar snap peas for 5 minutes.
- Serve with a sprinkle of scallions.

Nutrition:
Calories - 304
Protein - 9 g
Carbs - 38 g
Fat - 13 g
Sodium (Na) - 36 mg
Potassium (K) - 114 mg
Phosphorus - 101 mg

Baked Eggplant Tray

Preparation Time: 10 minutes
Cooking Time: 20 minutes
Servings: 2

Ingredients:
3 cups of eggplant
3 large omega-3 eggs
½ cup of liquid non-dairy creamer
1 teaspoon of vinegar
1 teaspoon of lemon juice
½ teaspoon of pepper
¼ teaspoon of sage
½ cup of white breadcrumbs
1 tablespoon of margarine

Directions:
➢ Preheat the oven to a temperature of about 350°F.
➢ Peel the eggplant and cut it into pieces.
➢ Place the eggplant pieces in a large pan; then cover it with water, and let boil until it becomes tender.
➢ Drain the eggplants and mash it very well.
➢ Combine the beaten eggs with non-dairy creamer, vinegar, lemon juice, pepper and sage with the mashed eggplant; then place it into a greased baking tray.
➢ Mix the melted margarine with the breadcrumbs.
➢ Top your tray with the breadcrumbs and bake it for about 20 minutes.
➢ Set the tray aside to cool for about 5 minutes.
➢ Serve and enjoy your dinner!

Nutrition:
Calories - 126
Fats - 8g
Carbs - 4.7g
Fiber - 1.6g
Potassium - 224mg
Sodium - 143mg
Phosphorous - 115g
Protein - 7.3g

Ciabatta Rolls with Chicken Pesto

Preparation Time: 10 minutes

Cooking Time: 20 minutes

Servings: 2

Ingredients:

6 teaspoon. of Greek yogurt

6 teaspoon. of pesto

2 small ciabatta rolls

8 oz. of shredded iceberg or romaine lettuce

8 oz. of cooked boneless and skinless chicken breast (shredded)

.125 teaspoon. of pepper

Directions:

➢ Combine the shredded chicken, pesto, pepper and Greek yogurt in a medium-sized bowl.

➢ Slice and toast the ciabatta rolls.

➢ Divide the shredded chicken and pesto mixture in half, and make sandwiches with the ciabatta rolls.

➢ Top with shredded lettuce if desired.

Nutrition:

Calories - 374

Fat - 10g

Carbs - 40g

Protein - 30g

Sodium - 522mg

Potassium - 360mg

Phosphorus - 84mg

Marinated Shrimp Pasta Salad

Preparation Time: 15 minutes

Cooking Time: 5 hours

Servings: 1

Ingredients:

¼ cup of honey

¼ cup of balsamic vinegar

½ English cucumber (cubed)

½ pound of fully cooked shrimp

15 baby carrots

1½ cups of dime-sized cut cauliflower

4 stalks of celery (diced)

½ large yellow bell pepper (diced)

½ red onion (diced)

½ large red bell pepper (diced)

12 ounces of uncooked tri-color pasta (cooked)

¾ cup of olive oil

3 teaspoon. of mustard (Dijon)

½ teaspoon. of garlic (powder)

½ teaspoon. of pepper

Directions:

➢ Cut vegetables and put them in a bowl with the shrimp.
➢ Whisk together the honey, balsamic vinegar, garlic powder, pepper and Dijon mustard in a small bowl. Add the oil and whisk it all together.
➢ Add pasta to the bowl with shrimp and vegetables, then mix it.
➢ Toss the sauce to coat the pasta, shrimp and vegetables evenly.
➢ Cover and chill for a minimum of five hours before serving.
➢ Stir and serve while chilled.

Nutrition:

Calories - 205

Fat - 13g

Carbs - 10g

Protein - 12g

Sodium - 363mg

Potassium - 156mg

Phosphorus - 109mg

Herby Beef Stroganoff and Fluffy Rice

Preparation Time: 15 minutes

Cooking Time: 5 hours

Servings: 6

Ingredients:

½ cup onion

2 garlic cloves

9 ounces of flat cut beef brisket, cut into 1" cubes

½ cup of low-sodium beef stock

⅓ cup of red wine

½ teaspoon of dried oregano

¼ teaspoon of freshly ground black pepper

½ teaspoon of dried thyme

½ teaspoon of saffron

½ cup of almond milk (unenriched)

¼ cup of all-purpose flour

1 cup of water

2 ½ cups of white rice

Directions:

➢ Chop up the onion and mince the garlic cloves.
➢ Mix the beef, stock, wine, onion, garlic, oregano, pepper, thyme and saffron in your slow cooker.
➢ Cover and cook on High until the beef is tender, for about 4 to 5 hours.
➢ Combine the almond milk, flour and water.
➢ Whisk together until smooth.
➢ Add the flour mixture to the slow cooker.
➢ Cook for another 15 to 25 minutes until the stroganoff is thick.
➢ Cook the rice using the package instructions, leaving out salt.
➢ Drain off the excess water.
➢ Serve the stroganoff over the rice.

Nutrition:

Calories – 241 Protein - 15g

Carbohydrates - 29g Fat - 5g

Cholesterol - 39g Sodium - 182mg

Potassium - 206mg Phosphorus - 151mg Calcium - 59mg

Chunky Beef and Potato Slow Roast

Preparation Time: 15 minutes

Cooking Time: 5 to 6 hours

Servings: 12

Ingredients:

3 cups of peeled potatoes (chunked)

1 cup of onion

2 garlic cloves (chopped)

1 ¼ pounds of flat cut beef brisket (fat trimmed)

2 of cups of water

1 teaspoon of chili powder

1 tablespoon of dried rosemary

Ingredients (for the sauce):

1 tablespoon of freshly grated horseradish

½ cup of almond milk (unenriched)

1 tablespoon of lemon juice (freshly squeezed)

1 garlic clove (minced)

A pinch of cayenne pepper

Directions:

➢ Double boil the potatoes to reduce their potassium content (hint: bring your potato to the boil, then drain and refill with water to boil again).

➢ Chop the onion and the garlic.

➢ Place the beef brisket in slow cooker.

➢ Combine water, chopped garlic, chili powder and rosemary.

➢ Pour the mixture over the brisket.

➢ Cover and cook on High for 4 to 5 hours until the meat is very tender.

➢ Drain the potatoes and add them to the slow cooker.

➢ Turn heat to High, and cook covered until the potatoes are tender.

➢ Prepare the horseradish sauce by whisking together horseradish, milk, lemon juice, minced garlic and cayenne pepper.

➢ Cover and refrigerate.

➢ Serve your casserole with a dash of horseradish sauce on the side.

Nutrition:

Calories – 199 Protein - 21g

Carbohydrates - 12g Fat - 7g Cholesterol - 63mg Sodium - 282mg

Potassium – 317 Phosphorus - 191mg Calcium - 23mg Fiber - 1g

Spiced Lamb Burgers

Preparation Time: 10 minutes

Cooking Time: 20 minutes

Servings: 2

Ingredients:

1 tablespoon of extra-virgin olive oil

1 teaspoon of cumin

½ finely diced red onion

1 minced garlic clove

1 teaspoon of harissa spices

1 cup of arugula

1 juiced lemon

6-ounce lean ground lamb

1 tablespoon of parsley

½ cup of low-fat plain yogurt

Directions:

➢ Preheat the broiler on a medium to high heat.
➢ Mix together the ground lamb, red onion, parsley, Harissa spices and olive oil until combined.
➢ Shape 1-inch thick patties using wet hands.
➢ Add the patties to a baking tray and place under the broiler for 7-8 minutes on each side, or until thoroughly cooked through.
➢ Mix the yogurt, lemon juice and cumin.
➢ Serve over the lamb burgers with a side salad of arugula.

Nutrition:

Calories - 306

Fat - 20g

Carbs - 10g

Phosphorus - 269mg

Potassium (K) - 492mg

Sodium (Na) - 86mg

Protein - 23g

Pork Loins with Leeks

Preparation Time: 10 minutes

Cooking Time: 35 minutes

Servings: 2

Ingredients:

1 sliced leek

1 tablespoon of mustard seeds

6-ounce Pork tenderloin

1 tablespoon of cumin seeds

1 tablespoon of dry mustard

1 tablespoon of extra-virgin oil

Directions:

➢ Preheat the broiler to medium high heat.

➢ In a dry skillet, heat mustard and cumin seeds until they start to pop (3 to 5 minutes).

➢ Grind seeds using pestle and mortar, or use a blender, then mix in the dry mustard.

➢ Coat the pork on both sides with the mustard blend, and add to a baking tray to broil for 25 to 30 minutes, or until cooked through. Turn once halfway through.

➢ Remove and place to one side.

➢ Heat the oil in a pan on medium heat, and add the leeks for 5 to 6 minutes, or until soft.

➢ Serve the pork tenderloin on a bed of leeks and enjoy!

Nutrition:

Calories - 139

Fat - 5g

Carbs - 2g

Phosphorus - 278mg

Potassium (K) - 45mg

Sodium (Na) - 47mg

Protein - 18g

Shrimp Szechuan

Preparation Time: 10 minutes

Cooking Time: 9 minutes

Servings: 4

Ingredients:

1 tablespoon of canola oil

½ cup of bean sprouts

½ cup of green bell pepper (chopped)

½ cup of onion (chopped)

½ cup of raw mushroom pieces

1 teaspoon of grated ginger root

½ teaspoon of garlic powder

1 tablespoon of sesame oil

1 teaspoon of red pepper flakes

⅓ cup of low-sodium chicken broth

4 tablespoons of sherry wine

1 teaspoon of cornstarch

4 oz. of frozen shrimp

Directions:

➢ Start by heating oil in the Instant pot on Sauté mode.

➢ Toss in onions, ginger, mushrooms, bell pepper and bean sprouts.

➢ Sauté for 2 minutes, then toss in all the other ingredients except cornstarch.

➢ Seal the lid and cook for 2 minutes on Manual mode at High pressure.

➢ Release the pressure completely, then remove the pot's lid once the cooking is done.

➢ Mix the cornstarch with 2 tablespoons of water in a bowl.

➢ Pour this mixture into the Instant pot, and cook for 5 minutes on sauté mode.

➢ Serve warm.

Nutrition:

Calories 140

Fats - 4.3g

Carbs - 6g

Fiber - 0.3g

Protein - 19g

Sodium - 372mg

Potassium - 204.3 mg

Phosphorus - 196mg

Shrimp & Broccoli

Preparation Time: 10 minutes

Cooking Time: 5 minutes

Servings: 4

Ingredients:

1 tablespoon of olive oil

1 clove of garlic (minced)

1 pound of shrimp

¼ cup of red bell pepper

1 cup of steamed broccoli florets

10 ounces of cream cheese

½ teaspoon of garlic powder

¼ cup of lemon juice

¾ teaspoon of ground peppercorns

¼ cup of half and half creamer

Directions:

- ➢ Pour the oil and cook the garlic for 30 seconds.
- ➢ Add shrimp and cook for 2 minutes.
- ➢ Add the rest of the ingredients.
- ➢ Mix well.
- ➢ Cook for 2 minutes.

Nutrition:

Calories - 469

Protein - 28 g

Carbohydrates - 28 g

Fat - 28 g

Cholesterol - 213 mg

Sodium - 374 mg

Potassium - 469 mg

Phosphorus - 335 mg

Calcium - 157 mg

Fiber - 2.6 g

Citrus Glazed Salmon

Preparation Time: 20 minutes

Cooking Time: 17 minutes

Servings: 4

Ingredients:

2 garlic cloves (crushed)

1 ½ tablespoons of lemon juice

2 tablespoons of olive oil

1 tablespoon of butter

1 tablespoon of Dijon mustard

2 dashes of cayenne pepper

1 teaspoon of dried basil leaves

1 teaspoon of dried dill

24 oz. of salmon filet

Directions:

> ➤ Place a 1-quart saucepan over moderate heat, and add oil, butter, garlic, lemon juice, mustard, cayenne pepper, dill, and basil to the pan.
> ➤ Stir this mixture for 5 minutes after it has boiled.
> ➤ Prepare and preheat a charcoal grill over moderate heat.
> ➤ Place the fish on a foil sheet and fold the edges to make a foil tray.
> ➤ Pour the prepared sauce over the fish.
> ➤ Place the fish in the foil in the preheated grill and cook for 12 minutes.
> ➤ Slice and serve.

Nutrition:

Calories - 401

Total Fat - 20.5g

Cholesterol - 144mg

Sodium - 256mg

Carbohydrate - 0.5g

Calcium - 549mg

Phosphorous - 214mg

Potassium - 446mg

Broiled Salmon Fillets

Preparation Time: 10 minutes

Cooking Time: 13 minutes

Servings: 4

Ingredients:

1 tablespoon of grated ginger root

1 clove of garlic (minced)

¼ cup of maple syrup

1 tablespoon of hot pepper sauce

4 salmon fillets (skinless)

Directions:

- ➢ Grease a pan with cooking spray and place it over moderate heat.
- ➢ Add ginger and garlic, then sauté for 3 minutes and transfer to a bowl.
- ➢ Add the hot pepper sauce and maple syrup to the ginger & garlic.
- ➢ Mix well, and keep this mixture aside.
- ➢ Place the salmon fillet in a suitable baking tray, greased with cooking oil.
- ➢ Brush the maple sauce over the fillets liberally.
- ➢ Broil them for 10 minutes in an oven at broiler settings.
- ➢ Serve warm.

Nutrition:

Calories - 289

Total Fat - 11.1g

Sodium - 80mg

Carbohydrate - 13.6g

Calcium - 78mg

Phosphorous - 230mg

Potassium - 331mg

Broiled Shrimp

Preparation Time: 10 minutes

Cooking Time: 5 minutes

Servings: 8

Ingredients:

1 lb. of shrimp in shell

½ cup of unsalted butter (melted)

2 teaspoons of lemon juice

2 tablespoons of chopped onion

1 clove of garlic (minced)

⅛ teaspoon of pepper

Directions:

➢ Toss the shrimp with the butter, lemon juice, onion, garlic and pepper in a bowl.

➢ Spread the seasoned shrimp in a baking tray.

➢ Broil for 5 minutes in an oven on broiler setting.

➢ Serve warm.

Nutrition:

Calories - 164

Total Fat - 12.8g

Sodium - 242mg

Carbohydrate - 0.6g

Calcium - 45mg

Phosphorous - 215mg

Potassium - 228mg

CHAPTER 13:

Side Dish Recipes

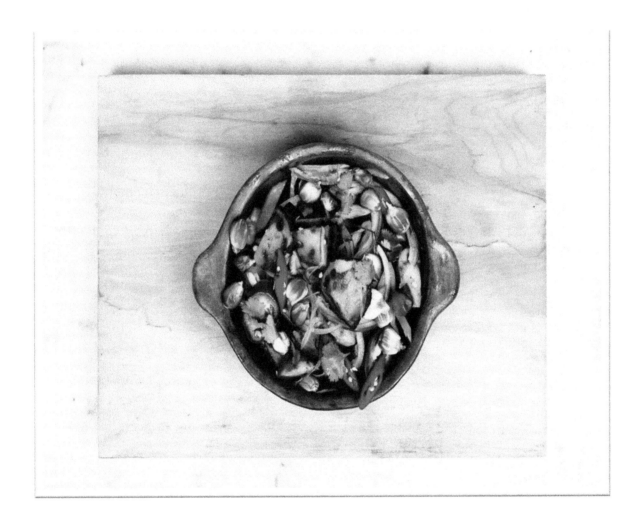

Crispy Parmesan Cauliflower

Preparation Time: 5 minutes
Cooking Time: 30 minutes
Servings: 2

Ingredients:
2 cups of Cauliflower florets -
.125 teaspoon of ground Black pepper
2 cloves of Garlic (minced)
2 tablespoons of grated Parmesan cheese
¼ cup of bread crumbs (plain)
1 tablespoon of olive oil

Directions:
➢ Preheat your oven to 400°F, and line a baking sheet with kitchen parchment.
➢ In one small bowl, combine olive oil and garlic.
➢ In another bowl, combine the Parmesan cheese, bread crumbs and black pepper.
➢ Dip the cauliflower piece-by-piece first into the olive oil mixture, and then into the bread crumb mixture.
➢ After you coat each piece, set it on the kitchen parchment-lined sheet.
➢ Place the cauliflower sheet in the middle of the oven and roast the cauliflower until it reaches golden brown perfection (about 30 minutes).
➢ Serve it immediately, while it is still warm and crispy.

Nutrition:
Calories - 106
Protein - 5g
Phosphorus - 166mg
Potassium - 369mg
Sodium - 222mg
Fat - 9g
Total Carbohydrates - 16g
Net Carbohydrates - 14g

Parmesan Quinoa with Peas

Preparation Time: 5 minutes

Cooking Time: 20 minutes

Servings: 2

Ingredients:

¾ cup of Quinoa -

1½ cups of Water

¾ cup of green peas (thawed if frozen)

¼ teaspoon of ground black pepper

1½ tablespoons of olive oil

3 tablespoons of grated Parmesan cheese

Directions:

➢ Place the uncooked quinoa in a fine metal sieve, and rinse it well with water until there is no debris running off.

➢ Place the quinoa and water in a metal saucepan, and bring it to a boil over medium heat.

➢ Once it begins to boil, reduce it to a light simmer, cover the pot with a lid, and continue cooking until all the water has been absorbed. This should take 15 to 20 minutes.

➢ Allow the quinoa to sit with the lid on for five minutes after turning off the heat.

➢ Once it's set, use a fork to fluff the quinoa, and stir in the green peas, olive oil and quinoa.

➢ Close the lid once again, allowing it to sit for five additional minutes to warm the peas and melt the cheese.

➢ Enjoy the quinoa while warm.

Nutrition:

Calories - 386

Protein - 13g

Phosphorus - 378mg

Potassium - 465mg

Sodium - 144mg

Fat - 16g

Total Carbohydrates - 47g

Net Carbohydrates - 41g

Mushroom Orzo

Preparation Time: 5 minutes
Cooking Time: 20 minutes
Servings: 2

Ingredients:
¾ cup of Orzo
1¼ cup of low-sodium chicken broth
4 ounces of diced Mushrooms
3 cloves of Garlic (minced)
1 tablespoon of dehydrated onion flakes
1 tablespoon of olive oil
¼ teaspoon of ground sage

Directions:
➢ Place the diced mushrooms, olive oil and garlic in a medium-sized metal saucepan, and allow them to sauté over medium heat for five minutes.
➢ Add in the sage, onion flakes, orzo and low-sodium chicken broth.
➢ Bring the mixture to a boil.
➢ Reduce the heat of the skillet to a light simmer, cover the pot with a lid, and allow it to cook until all of the liquid has been absorbed (in about 9 minutes).
➢ Fluff the orzo with a fork before serving.

Nutrition:
Calories - 337
Protein - 18g
Phosphorus - 63mg
Potassium - 430mg
Sodium - 43mg
Fat - 8g
Total Carbohydrates - 99g
Net Carbohydrates - 95g

Cucumber Dill Salad with Greek Yogurt Dressing

Preparation Time: 5 minutes

Cooking Time: 0 minute

Servings: 2

Ingredients:

2 Cucumbers (cut thinly)

½ small red onion (thinly sliced)

3 tablespoons of plain Greek yogurt

2 teaspoons of honey

4 teaspoons of white vinegar

.125 teaspoon of ground black pepper

.125 teaspoon of garlic powder

1½ tablespoons of fresh Dill (chopped)

Directions:

➤ Use either a knife or a mandolin to cut the cucumbers into thin, even slices (about ¼ inch thick).

➤ In a medium bowl, whisk together the fresh dill, garlic powder, black pepper, white vinegar, honey and Greek yogurt.

➤ Into the bowl with the prepared Greek yogurt dressing, add the cucumbers and red onion; then toss them together until fully coated.

➤ Cover the bowl with a lid or plastic wrap, and allow it to chill in the fridge for at least an hour before enjoying (you can make this salad up to a day in advance).

Nutrition:

Calories - 106

Protein - 5g

Phosphorus - 166mg

Potassium - 369mg

Sodium - 222mg

Fat - 9g

Total Carbohydrates - 16g

Net Carbohydrates - 14g

Zesty Green Beans with Almonds

Preparation Time: 5 minutes

Cooking Time: 10 minutes

Servings: 2

Ingredients:

½ pound of trimmed green beans

1 tablespoon of olive oil

1 Shallot (diced)

2 cloves of Garlic (minced)

2 tablespoons of sliced Almonds

¼ teaspoon of lemon zest

1 teaspoon of lemon juice

.125 teaspoon of ground black pepper

Directions:

➢ In a large skillet, sauté the shallot and garlic in olive oil, over medium heat until soft (in about three minutes).

➢ Add in green beans and black pepper; then continue to cook the green beans until they are tender (in about seven minutes).

➢ Once the green beans are ready, stir in the lemon juice and lemon zest; then top the skillet off with the sliced almonds.

Nutrition:

Calories - 143

Protein - 3g

Phosphorus - 84mg

Potassium - 322mg

Sodium - 8mg

Fat - 10g

Total Carbohydrates - 11g

Net Carbohydrates - 8g

Almond Pasta Salad

Preparation Time: 10 minutes

Cooking Time: 10 minutes

Servings: 6

Ingredients:

1 lb. of cooked elbow macaroni

½ cup of sun-dried tomatoes (diced)

1 (15 oz.) can of make whole artichokes (diced)

1 orange bell pepper (diced)

3 green onions (sliced)

2 tablespoons of basil (sliced)

2 oz. of slivered almonds

Dressing:

1 garlic clove (minced)

1 tablespoon of Dijon mustard

1 tablespoon of raw honey

¼ cup of white balsamic vinegar

⅓ cup of olive oil

Directions:

> ➤ Preheat the oven to 350°F.
> ➤ Lay the almonds on a baking sheet and bake until golden brown.
> ➤ Cook the pasta according to the package instruction.
> ➤ Move to a serving bowl, and start tossing all the ingredients.
> ➤ Mix well and serve.

Nutrition:

Calories - 260

Fat - 7.7g

Sodium - 143mg

Phosphorus - 39mg

Potassium - 585mg

Carbohydrate - 41.4g

Protein - 9.6g

Pineapple Berry Salad

Preparation Time: 10 minutes

Cooking Time: 5 minutes

Servings: 4

Ingredients:

4 cups of pineapple (peeled & cubed)

3 cups of chopped strawberries

¼ cup of honey

½ cup of basil leaves

1 tablespoon of lemon zest

½ cup of blueberries

Directions:

➢ Prepare a salad bowl.

➢ Put all the ingredients.

➢ Mix well and serve.

Nutrition:

Calories - 128

Fat - 0.6g

Sodium - 3mg

Phosphorous - 151mg

Potassium - 362mg

Carbohydrate - 33.1g

Protein - 1.8g

Cabbage Pear Salad

Preparation Time: 15 minutes

Cooking Time: 1 hour

Servings: 6

Ingredients:

2 scallions (chopped)

2 cups of finely shredded green cabbage

1 cup of finely shredded red cabbage

½ red bell pepper (boiled & chopped)

½ cup of chopped cilantro

2 celery stalks (chopped)

1 Asian pear (cored and grated)

¼ cup of olive oil

Juice of 1 lime

Zest of 1 lime

1 teaspoon of granulated sugar

Directions:

➤ In a mixing bowl, add cabbages, scallions, celery, pear, red pepper and cilantro.

➤ Combine to mix well with each other.

➤ Take another mixing bowl; add olive oil, lime juice, lime zest and sugar. Then mix thoroughly.

➤ Add dressing over and toss well.

➤ Refrigerate for 1 hour; serve chilled.

Nutrition:

Calories - 128

Fat - 8g

Sodium - 57mg

Potassium - 149mg

Phosphorus - 25mg

Carbohydrates - 2g

Protein - 6g

Vegetables with Apple Juice

Preparation Time: 10 minutes

Cooking Time: 50 minutes

Servings: 4

Ingredients:

3 tablespoons of olive oil

3 cups of apple juice

1¼ pounds of turnips

1¼ pounds of carrots

1¼ pounds of cauliflower

Salt and pepper to taste

Directions:

➢ Boil apple juice in a large saucepan until reduced to ¾ cup (in about 30 minutes), then whisk in olive oil.

➢ Preheat oven to 425°F.

➢ Peel and cut vegetables into ½-inch pieces. Divide between 2 roasting pans.

➢ Pour apple juice mixture over vegetables; Sprinkle with salt and pepper; Toss to coat.

➢ Roast until vegetables are tender and golden, occasionally stirring (about 40 minutes).

Nutrition:

Calories - 91

Fat - 4.4g

Sodium - 19mg

Potassium - 215mg

Phosphorus - 150 mg

Carbohydrate - 13.3g

Dietary Fiber - 1.5g

Protein - 0.5g

Creamy Mushroom Peas

Preparation Time: 3 minutes

Cooking Time: 5 minutes

Servings: 4

Ingredients:

2 cups of frozen green peas

2 tablespoons of olive oil

1 cup of sliced fresh mushrooms

1 small chopped onion

1 tablespoon of all-purpose flour

¼ teaspoon of ground black pepper

1 pinch of ground cinnamon

Directions:

➢ Prepare a small saucepan with one inch of water. Boil it, then add peas.
➢ Cook until tender (in about 5 minutes), then drain and set aside.
➢ Add mushrooms and onions in a medium saucepan, cook for a few minutes, or until it becomes tender.
➢ Sprinkle flour over the mushrooms, cook for 1 minute, and season with pepper and cinnamon while constantly stirring.
➢ Cook, stirring until smooth and thick. Stir in peas and remove from heat.
➢ Let it stand for 5 minutes before serving.

Nutrition:

Calories - 128

Fat - 6.1g

Sodium - 46mg

Potassium - 264mg

Phosphorus - 45 mg

Carbohydrate - 14.3g

Dietary Fiber - 4.4g

Protein - 4.9g

Stir-Fried Beans and Mushrooms

Preparation Time: 5 minutes

Cooking Time: 10 minutes

Servings: 4

Ingredients:

1 tablespoon of olive oil

½ pound of green beans

4 ounces of fresh thinly sliced mushrooms

1 teaspoon of black pepper

Directions:

- ➤ Heat oil in skillet over medium to high heat.
- ➤ Stir in green beans and mushrooms, then cook for 3 to 4 minutes, until it's tender.
- ➤ Transfer beans and mushrooms to a medium bowl.
- ➤ Toss with black pepper and serve warm.

Nutrition:

Calories - 43

Fat - 3.6g

Sodium - 1mg

Potassium - 56mg

Phosphorus - 48mg

Carbohydrate - 2.1g

Dietary Fiber - 0.7g

Protein - 1.1g

Celery Salad

Preparation Time: 10 minutes

Cooking Time: 0 minutes

Servings: 4

Ingredients:

1 cup of sliced celery

⅓ cup of dried sweet cherries

⅓ cup of frozen green peas (thawed)

3 tablespoons of chopped fresh basil

1 tablespoon of chopped macadamia nuts (toasted)

1½ tablespoons of fat-free mayonnaise

1½ teaspoons of fresh lemon juice

⅛ teaspoon of salt

⅛ teaspoon of ground black pepper

Directions:

➢ Combine the celery, cherries, peas, basil, and macadamia nuts in a small bowl.
➢ Stir in the mayonnaise and lemon juice.
➢ Season with salt and pepper.
➢ Chill before serving.

Nutrition:

Calories - 56

Fat - 3.1g

Sodium - 135mg

Potassium - 121mg

Phosphorus - 98mg

Carbohydrate - 5.9g

Dietary Fiber - 1.3g

Protein - 1.5g

Beans with Basil

Preparation Time: 5 minutes

Cooking Time: 5 minutes

Servings: 4

Ingredients:

2 teaspoons of butter

¾ pounds of green beans (trimmed)

3 green onions (chopped)

1 clove of garlic (chopped)

⅛ teaspoon of salt

⅛ teaspoon of pepper

1 tablespoon of chopped fresh basil

Directions:

➤ Ready a large skillet and melt the butter over medium heat.

➤ Add the beans, green onion, garlic, salt and pepper.

➤ Sauté for 4 minutes, then remove from heat and stir in the basil leaves.

Nutrition:

Calories - 21

Total Fat - 1.3g

Sodium - 61mg

Potassium - 58mg

Phosphorus - 40mg

Carbohydrate - 2g

Dietary Fiber - 0.7g

Protein - 0.7g

Green Pea Patties

Preparation Time: 10 minutes

Cooking Time: 15 minutes

Servings: 4

Ingredients:

½ pound of green peas

½ cup of all-purpose flour

1 egg white

1 tablespoon of soy milk (or as needed)

1 teaspoon of baking powder

⅛ teaspoon of salt

⅛ teaspoon of ground black pepper to taste

1 tablespoon of olive oil (or as needed)

Directions:

➢ Prepare a large pot of water and let it boil.

➢ Cook peas in the boiling water, and stir until tender.

➢ Drain and move to a bowl; then mash it is using a fork.

➢ Mix flour, egg white, milk, baking powder and pepper into mashed peas. You can add more milk or flour until the mixture holds together.

➢ Shape the mixture into patties.

➢ Cook the patties over medium heat 3 to 4 minutes per side, or until golden.

Nutrition:

Calories - 91

Fat - 3.5g

Sodium - 24mg

Potassium - 140mg

Phosphorus - 124mg

Carbohydrate - 11.7g

Dietary Fiber - 1.1g

Protein - 3.6g

Peas and Cauliflower

Preparation Time: 10 minutes

Cooking Time: 20 minutes

Servings: 4

Ingredients:

3 tablespoons of olive oil

4 teaspoons of cumin seed

1 teaspoon of mustard seed

2 cups of green peas

2 cups of cauliflower florets

⅛ teaspoon of salt

⅛ teaspoon of pepper

Directions:

➢ Put the cumin and mustard seeds in hot oil.
➢ Cook until the seeds begin to pop.
➢ Mix in the peas and cauliflower, then season with salt.
➢ Continue cooking for 15 minutes until the vegetables are tender.

Nutrition:

Calories - 78

Fat - 4.4g

Sodium - 87mg

Potassium - 208mg

Phosphorus - 148mg

Carbohydrate - 7.8g

Dietary Fiber - 2.8g

Protein - 3.1g

Mashed Peas

Preparation Time: 5 minutes
Cooking Time: 10 minutes
Servings: 4

Ingredients:
2 tablespoons of olive oil
1 cup of green peas
1 bunch of fresh mint leaves
1 bunch of green onions (chopped)
2 tablespoons of honey
Salt and pepper to taste

Directions:
- Prepare skillet and stir the peas, mint leaves and green onions in heated olive oil until the peas are tender (in7 to 10 minutes).
- Put the peas into a bowl and mash until the peas are thoroughly crushed but still slightly chunky.
- Add honey, salt and pepper; then mix until the honey mixed well.
- Serve warm or cold.

Nutrition:
Calories - 83
Fat - 4.8g
Sodium - 2mg
Potassium - 78mg
Phosphorus - 48mg
Carbohydrate - 9.6g
Dietary Fiber - 1.5g
Protein - 1.4g

Stuffed Zucchini Boats

Preparation Time: 15 minutes

Cooking Time: 20 minutes

Servings: 4

Ingredients:

2 medium zucchinis

4 slices of white bread

¼ teaspoon of ground sage

1 teaspoon of onion powder

¼ teaspoon of dried basil

1 teaspoon of salt-free lemon pepper

1 teaspoon of dill weed

Directions:

➢ Pre-heat oven to 375°F.
➢ Slice the zucchini in half lengthwise.
➢ Remove seeds using a spoon, forming a trench in each zucchini half.
➢ Boil zucchini for 3 to 5 minutes.
➢ Toast two slices of bread while zucchini is cooking.
➢ Put the toast and two uncooked pieces of bread in a food processor to make breadcrumbs.
➢ Add seasonings and mix the breadcrumbs well.
➢ Add the zucchini and water, then blend with a fork to get stuffing consistency.
➢ Remove zucchini from water and place in baking dish; peel side down.
➢ Spoon stuffing into a trench in each zucchini half.
➢ Bake for 20 minutes and serve.

Nutrition:

Calories - 42

Fat - 0.5g

Sodium - 72mg

Potassium - 283mg

Phosphorus - 63mg

Carbohydrate - 8.5g

Dietary Fiber - 1.4g

Protein - 2g

CHAPTER 14:

Dessert Recipes

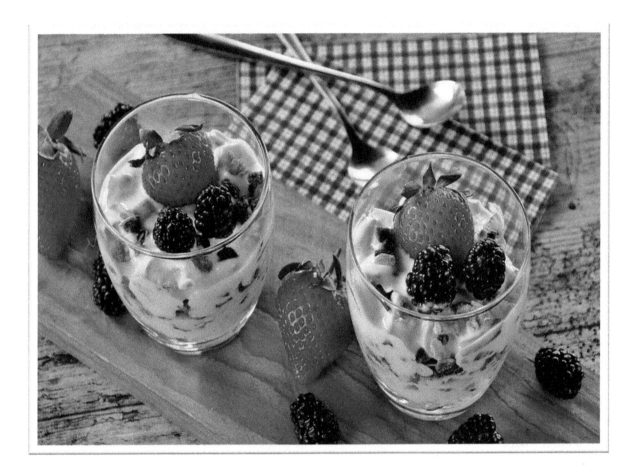

Maple Crisp Bars

Preparation Time: 5 minutes

Cooking Time: 5 minutes

Servings: 20

Ingredients:

⅓ cup of butter

1 cup of brown Swerve

1 teaspoon of maple extract

½ cup of maple syrup

8 cups of puffed rice cereal

Directions:

➢ Mix the butter with Swerve, maple extract and syrup in a saucepan over moderate heat.

➢ Cook by slowly stirring this mixture for 5 minutes, then toss in the rice cereal.

➢ Mix well, then press this cereal mixture in a 13x9 inches baking dish.

➢ Refrigerate the mixture for 2 hours, then cut into 20 bars.

➢ Serve.

Nutrition:

Calories - 107

Total Fat - 3.1g

Saturated Fat - 0.5g

Cholesterol - 0mg

Sodium - 36mg

Carbohydrate - 10.6g

Dietary Fiber - 0.1g

Sugars - 5.4g

Protein - 0.4g

Calcium - 7mg

Phosphorous - 233mg

Potassium - 24mg

Apple Pie

Preparation Time: 10 minutes

Cooking Time: 50 minutes

Servings: 6

Ingredients:

6 medium apples (peeled, cored & sliced)

½ cup of granulated sugar

1 teaspoon of ground cinnamon

6 tablespoons of butter

2⅔ cups of all-purpose flour

1 cup of shortening

6 tablespoons of water

Directions:

➢ Preheat your oven to 425°F.

➢ Toss the apple slices with cinnamon and sugar in a bowl, then cover and set it aside.

➢ Blend the flour with the shortening in a pastry blender, then add chilled water by the tablespoon.

➢ Continue mixing and adding the water until it forms a smooth dough ball.

➢ Divide the dough into two equal-size pieces, and spread them into 2 separate 9-inch sheets.

➢ Arrange the sheet of dough at the bottom of a 9-inch pie pan.

➢ Spread the apples in the pie shell and spread a tablespoon of butter over it.

➢ Cover the filling with the remaining sheet of the dough, and pinch down the edges.

➢ Carve 1-inch cuts on top of the pie, and bake for 50 minutes or more until golden.

➢ Slice and serve.

Nutrition:

Calories - 517

Protein - 4g

Carbohydrates - 51g

Fat - 33g

Cholesterol - 24mg

Sodium - 65mg

Potassium - 145mg

Phosphorus - 43mg

Calcium - 24mg

Fiber - 2.7g

Banana Pudding Dessert

Preparation Time: 10 minutes

Cooking Time: 5 minutes

Servings: 4

Ingredients:

12 oz. of vanilla wafers

2 boxes of banana cream pudding mix

2½ cups of unenriched rice milk

8 oz. of dairy whipped topping

Directions:

> ➢ Line the bottom of a 9x13 inch pan with a layer of wafers.
> ➢ Mix the banana pudding mix with 2½ cups of milk in a saucepan.
> ➢ Bring it to a boil while constantly stirring.
> ➢ Pour the banana pudding over the wafers.
> ➢ Add another layer of wafers over the pudding layer and press them down gently.
> ➢ Place the layered pudding in the refrigerator for 1 hour.
> ➢ Garnish with whipped cream and serve.

Nutrition:

Calories - 259

Protein - 3g

Carbohydrates - 46g

Fat - 7g

Cholesterol - 3mg

Sodium - 276mg

Potassium - 52mg

Phosphorus - 40mg

Calcium - 9mg

Fiber - 0.3g

Strawberry Pizza

Preparation Time: 10 minutes
Cooking Time: 15 minutes
Servings: 12

Ingredients (crust):
1 cup of flour
¼ cup of Swerve
½ cup of butter

Ingredients (filling):
8 oz. of softened cream cheese
½ teaspoon of vanilla
¾ tablespoon of stevia
2 cups of sliced strawberries

Directions:
- Mix the flour with the Swerve, butter and enough water to make a dough.
- Spread this dough evenly in a pie pan.
- Bake the crust for 15 minutes at 350°F.
- Beat the cream cheese with the stevia and vanilla in a mixer until fluffy.
- Spread this cream cheese filling in the crust and top it with strawberries.
- Serve.

Nutrition:
Calories - 235
Total Fat - 14.5g
Saturated Fat - 9g
Cholesterol - 41mg
Sodium - 112mg
Carbohydrate - 12.8g
Dietary Fiber - 1g
Sugars - 9.3g
Protein - 2.8g
Calcium - 25mg
Phosphorous - 236mg
Potassium - 84mg

Pumpkin Cinnamon Roll

Preparation Time: 8 minutes

Cooking Time: 15 minutes

Servings: 24

Ingredients (dough):

1½ cups of milk

½ cup of olive oil

½ cup of granulated Swerve

2¼ teaspoons of active dry yeast

1 cup of pumpkin puree

4½ cups of flour

½ teaspoon of ground cinnamon

¼ teaspoon of ground ginger

¼ teaspoon of ground nutmeg

½ teaspoon of baking powder

½ teaspoon of baking soda

Melted butter (for buttering pans)

Ingredients (filling):

½ cup of butter (melted)

½ cup of brown Swerve

½ cup of granulated Swerve

½ teaspoon of cinnamon

½ teaspoon of ground ginger

¼ teaspoon of ground nutmeg

Directions:

> ➢ Switch on your gas oven and let it preheat at 375°F.
> ➢ Whisk all the ingredients for the dough in a mixing bowl.
> ➢ Spread the dough in a loaf pan into a ½-inch layer, and bake it for 15 minutes.
> ➢ Meanwhile, whisk all the ingredients for the filling in a bowl.
> ➢ Place the baked cake in a serving plate and top it with the prepared filling.
> ➢ Roll the cake and slice it. Serve.

Nutrition:

Calories – 201 Total Fat - 9.2g Saturated Fat - 3.7g

Cholesterol - 12mg Sodium - 63mg Carbohydrate - 14.9g Dietary Fiber - 1g

Sugars - 3.1g Protein - 3.2g Calcium - 32mg Phosphorous - 277mg Potassium - 91mg

Blueberry Cream Cones

Preparation Time: 10 minutes

Cooking Time: 0 minutes

Total time: 10 minutes

Servings: 6

Ingredients:

4 oz. of cream cheese

1½ cup of whipped topping

1¼ cup of fresh or frozen blueberries

¼ cup of blueberry jam or preserves

6 small ice cream cones

Directions:

➢ Start by softening the cream cheese, then beat it in a mixer until fluffy.

➢ Fold in jam and fruits.

➢ Divide the mixture into the ice cream cones.

➢ Serve fresh.

Nutrition:

Calories - 177

Protein - 3g

Carbohydrates - 21g

Fat - 9g

Cholesterol - 21mg

Sodium - 95mg

Potassium - 81mg

Phosphorus - 40mg

Calcium - 24mg

Fiber - 1.0g

Cherry Coffee Cake

Preparation Time: 10 minutes
Cooking Time: 40 minutes
Servings: 6

Ingredients:
½ cup of unsalted butter
2 eggs
1 cup of granulated sugar
1 cup of sour cream
1 teaspoon vanilla
2 cups of all-purpose white flour
1 teaspoon of baking powder
1 teaspoon of baking soda
20 oz. of cherry pie filling

Directions:
➢ Preheat oven to 350°F.
➢ Soften the butter first, then beat it with the eggs, sugar, vanilla and sour cream in a mixer.
➢ Separately mix flour with baking soda and baking powder.
➢ Add this mixture to the egg mixture, and mix well until smooth.
➢ Spread this batter evenly in a 9x13 inch baking pan.
➢ Bake the pie for 40 minutes in the oven until golden on the surface.
➢ Slice and serve with cherry pie filling on top.

Nutrition:
Calories - 204
Protein - 3g
Carbohydrates - 30g
Fat - 8g
Cholesterol - 43mg
Sodium - 113mg
Potassium - 72mg
Phosphorus - 70mg
Calcium - 41mg
Fiber - 0.5g

Grilled Peach Sundaes

Preparation Time: 5 minutes

Cooking Time: 0 minute

Servings: 1

Ingredients:

1 tablespoon of toasted unsweetened coconut

1 teaspoon of canola oil

2 peaches (halved and pitted)

2 scoops of non-fat vanilla yogurt (frozen)

Directions:

➢ Brush the peaches with oil, and grill until tender.

➢ Place peach halves on a bowl and top with frozen yogurt and coconut.

Nutrition:

Calories - 61

Carbs - 2g

Protein - 2g

Fats - 6g

Phosphorus - 32mg

Potassium - 85mg

Sodium - 30mg

Belgian Waffle with Fruits

Preparation Time: 10 minutes

Cooking Time: 25 minutes

Servings: 6

Ingredients:

2 large Eggs

2 cups of Cake flour

¾ teaspoon of baking soda

¾ cup of sour cream

¾ cup of 1% low-fat milk

2 teaspoons of vanilla extract

4 tablespoons of unsalted butter

2 tablespoons of granulated sugar

6 tablespoons of powdered sugar

Directions:

- ➤ Start by heating the waffle iron.
- ➤ Now take a large mixing bowl, then add in the baking soda and cake flour. Mix these well and set aside.
- ➤ Take 2 medium bowls and separate the egg whites from the yolks.
- ➤ Add the vanilla extract and sour cream to the bowl with the egg yolks, and whisk well.
- ➤ Add the melted butter and mix well.
- ➤ Take the second bowl with the egg whites. Using a mixer on medium speed, beat the eggs to form soft peaks.
- ➤ Add in granulated sugar and beat for another 3 to 4 minutes to form stiff peaks.
- ➤ Whisk together the flour mixture and sour cream mixture to combine well.
- ➤ Add in the egg white mixture and gently fold through.
- ➤ Add approximately ½ cup of batter to the heated waffle iron and close the iron.
- ➤ Cook the mixture for 3 minutes. Once done, empty onto a serving platter.
- ➤ Garnish with powdered sugar, fresh berries, syrup and whipped cream.

Nutrition:

Carbohydrates - 50g Protein - 8g

Fat - 15g Sodium - 204mg

Cholesterol - 98mg

Potassium - 151mg

Calcium - 81mg

Phosphorus - 121mg Fiber - 1g

Spicy Broccoli Macaroni

Preparation Time: 10 minutes

Cooking Time: 25 minutes

Servings: 2

Ingredients:

1 cup of boiled macaroni

2 teaspoons of garlic (chopped)

½ teaspoon of red chilies (chopped)

¼ cup of broccoli

Pepper

Olive oil

Directions:

 ➢ Heat oil in a pan and sauté the garlic.
 ➢ Add red chilies. Season with salt and pepper.
 ➢ Add broccoli and cook for two minutes.
 ➢ Add boiled macaroni.
 ➢ Cook for 2 to 3 minutes, and serve hot.

Nutrition:

Calories - 102

Total Fat - 4.6g

Saturated Fat - 1.1g

Cholesterol - 3mg

Sodium - 35mg

Total Carbohydrate - 11.9g

Dietary Fiber - 0.8g

Total Sugar - 0.3g

Protein - 3.4g

Calcium - 39mg

Iron - 0mg

Potassium - 39mg

Phosphorus - 10 mg

Quick Quiche

Preparation Time: 15 minutes

Cooking Time: 35 minutes

Servings: 2

Ingredients:

1 teaspoon of olive oil

1 egg white (beaten)

1 tablespoon of finely chopped onion

¼ teaspoon of black pepper

¼ cup of all-purpose flour

½ cup of soy milk

Directions:

➤ Preheat oven to 350°F; then lightly grease a 9-inch pie pan.
➤ Combine egg white, olive oil, onion, black pepper, flour and soy milk; whisk together until smooth; pour into pie pan.
➤ Bake in preheated oven for 30 to 35 minutes, until set.
➤ Serve hot or cold.

Nutrition:

Calories - 121

Total Fat - 3.6g

Saturated Fat - 0.5g

Cholesterol - 0mg

Sodium - 48mg

Total Carbohydrate - 16.5g

Dietary Fiber - 1g

Total Sugar - 2.8g

Protein - 5.5g

Calcium - 21mg

Iron - 1mg

Potassium - 126mg

Phosphorus - 90 mg

Chocolate Trifle

Preparation Time: 20 minutes

Cooking Time: 15 minutes

Servings: 4

Ingredients:

1 small plain sponge swiss roll

3 oz. of custard powder

5 oz. of hot water

16 oz. of canned mandarins

3 tablespoons of sherry

5 oz. of double cream

4 chocolate squares (grated)

Directions:

 ➢ Whisk the custard powder with water in a bowl until dissolved.
 ➢ In a bowl, mix the custard well until it becomes creamy, and let it sit for 15 minutes.
 ➢ Spread the swiss roll and cut it in 4 squares.
 ➢ Place the swiss roll in the 4 serving cups.
 ➢ Top the swiss roll with mandarin, custard, cream and chocolate.
 ➢ Serve.

Nutrition:

Calories - 315

Total Fat - 13.5g

Cholesterol - 43mg

Sodium - 185mg

Protein - 2.9g

Calcium - 61mg

Phosphorous - 184mg

Potassium - 129mg

Cherry Dessert

Preparation Time: 10 minutes

Cooking Time: 20 minutes

Total time: 30 minutes

Servings: 6

Ingredients:

1 small package of sugar-free cherry gelatin

1 pie crust (9-inch size)

8 oz. of light cream cheese

12 oz. of whipped topping

20 oz. of cherry pie filling

Directions:

- ➢ Prepare the cherry gelatin according to the given instructions on the packet.
- ➢ Pour the mixture in an 8x8 inch pan and refrigerate until set.
- ➢ Soften the cream cheese at room temperature.
- ➢ Place the 9-inch pie crust in a pie pan and bake it until golden brown.
- ➢ Vigorously beat the cream cheese in a mixer until fluffy, and fold in whipped topping.
- ➢ Dice the gelatin into cubes, and add them to the cream cheese mixture.
- ➢ Mix gently, then add this mixture to the baking pie shell.
- ➢ Top the cream cheese filling with cherry pie filling.
- ➢ Refrigerate for 3 hours then slice to serve.

Nutrition:

Calories - 258

Protein - 5g

Carbohydrates - 28g

Fat - 13g

Cholesterol - 11mg

Sodium - 214mg

Potassium - 150mg

Phosphorus - 50mg

Calcium - 30mg

Fiber - 1.0g

Crunchy Peppermint Cookies

Preparation Time: 10 minutes

Cooking Time: 12 minutes

Servings: 6

Ingredients:

½ cup of unsalted butter

18 peppermint candies

¾ cup of sugar

1 large egg

¼ teaspoon of peppermint extract

1½ cups of all-purpose flour

1 teaspoon of baking powder

Directions:

➢ Soften the butter at room temperature.

➢ Add 12 peppermint candies to a ziplock bag and crush them using a mallet.

➢ Beat butter with egg, sugar and peppermint extract in a mixer until fluffy.

➢ Stir in baking powder and flour; then mix well until smooth.

➢ Stir in crushed peppermint candies and refrigerate the dough for 1 hour.

➢ Meanwhile, layer a baking sheet with parchment paper.

➢ Preheat the oven to 350°F.

➢ Crush the remaining candies and keep them aside.

➢ Make ¾ inch balls out of the dough and place them on the baking sheet.

➢ Sprinkle the crushed candies over the balls.

➢ Bake them for 12 minutes until slightly browned.

➢ Serve fresh and enjoy.

Nutrition:

Calories - 150

Protein - 2g

Carbohydrates - 22g

Fat - 6g

Cholesterol - 24mg

Sodium - 67mg

Potassium - 17mg

Phosphorus - 24mg

Calcium - 20mg

Fiber - 0.2g

Cranberries Snow

Preparation Time: 10 minutes

Cooking Time: 12 minutes

Servings: 4

Ingredients:

1 cup of cran-cherry juice

12 oz. of fresh cranberries

2 packets of gelatin

2 cups of granulated sugar

1 cup of crushed pineapple (canned in juice)

8 oz. of cream cheese

3 cups of whipped topping

Directions:

- ➤ Boil the cran-cherry juice in a saucepan.
- ➤ Stir in cranberries and cook for 12 minutes.
- ➤ Remove the pan from the stove heat, and add 1¼ cup of sugar and gelatin.
- ➤ Mix well until dissolved, then allow it to cool for 30 minutes.
- ➤ Toss in drained pineapple and mix well; then pour it all into a 9x13 inch pan.
- ➤ Refrigerate this mixture for 1 hour.
- ➤ Prepare the snow topping by mixing the ¾ sugar and cream cheese in a mixer.
- ➤ Spread this mixture over the refrigerated cranberry mixture.
- ➤ Serve fresh.

Nutrition:

Calories - 210

Protein - 2g

Carbohydrates - 35g

Fat - 7g

Cholesterol - 23mg

Sodium - 58mg

Potassium - 65mg

Phosphorus - 25mg

Calcium - 28mg

Fiber - 1.0g

Pineapple Gelatin Pie

Preparation Time: 10 minutes

Cooking Time: 5 minutes

Servings: 8

Ingredients:

⅔ cup of graham cracker crumbs

2½ tablespoons of melted butter

1 (20-oz) can of crushed pineapple (juice packed)

1 small gelatin pack

1 tablespoon of lemon juice

2 egg whites (pasteurized)

¼ teaspoon of cream of tartar

Directions:

➢ Whisk the crumbs with butter in a bowl, then spread them onto an 8-inch pie plate.

➢ Bake the crust for 5 minutes at 425°F.

➢ Meanwhile, mix the pineapple juice with gelatin in a saucepan.

➢ Place it over low heat, then add the pineapple and lemon juice. Mix well.

➢ Beat the cream of tartar and egg whites in a mixer until creamy.

➢ Add the cooked pineapple mixture, then mix well.

➢ Spread this filling in the baked crust.

➢ Refrigerate the pie for 4 hours, then slice.

➢ Serve.

Nutrition:

Calories - 106

Total Fat - 4.2g

Saturated Fat - 0.6g

Cholesterol - 0mg

Sodium - 117mg

Carbohydrate - 14.5g

Dietary Fiber - 0.5g

Sugars - 9.4g

Protein - 2.2g

Calcium - 3mg

Phosphorous - 231mg

Potassium - 33mg

Buttery Lemon Squares

Preparation Time: 5 minutes

Cooking Time: 35 minutes

Servings: 12

Ingredients:

1 cup of refined Swerve

1 cup of flour

½ cup of unsalted butter

1 cup of granulated Swerve

½ teaspoon of baking powder

2 eggs (beaten)

4 tablespoons of lemon juice

1 tablespoon of butter (unsalted, softened)

1 tablespoon of lemon zest

Directions:

➢ Start mixing ¼ cup of refined Swerve, ½ cup of butter and flour in a bowl.
➢ Spread this crust mixture in an 8-inche square pan and press it.
➢ Bake this flour crust for 15 minutes at 350°F.
➢ Meanwhile, prepare the filling by beating 2 tablespoons of lemon juice, granulated Swerve, eggs, lemon rind and baking powder in a mixer.
➢ Spread this filling in the baked crust, and bake again for about 20 minutes.
➢ Meanwhile, prepare the squares' icing by beating 2 tablespoons of lemon juice, 1 tablespoon of butter and ¾ cup of refine Swerve.
➢ Once the lemon pie is baked well, allow it to cool.
➢ Sprinkle the icing mixture on top of the lemon pie, then cut it into 36 squares. Serve.

Nutrition:

Calories – 229 Total Fat - 9.5g

Saturated Fat - 5.8g

Cholesterol - 50mg

Sodium - 66mg

Carbohydrate - 22.8g

Dietary Fiber - 0.3g

Sugars - 16g Protein - 2.1g

Calcium - 18mg Phosphorous - 257mg Potassium - 51mg

Chocolate Gelatin Mousse

Preparation Time: 5 minutes

Cooking Time: 5 minutes

Servings: 4

Ingredients:

1 teaspoon of stevia

½ teaspoon of gelatin

¼ cup of milk

½ cup of chocolate chips

1 teaspoon of vanilla

½ cup of heavy cream (whipped)

Directions:

➢ Whisk the stevia with gelatin and milk in a saucepan, and cook up to a boil.

➢ Stir in the chocolate and vanilla, then mix well until it has completely melted.

➢ Beat the cream in a mixer until fluffy, then fold in the chocolate mixture.

➢ Mix it gently with a spatula, then transfer to the serving bowl.

➢ Refrigerate the dessert for 4 hours.

➢ Serve.

Nutrition:

Calories - 200

Total Fat - 12.1g

Saturated Fat - 8g

Cholesterol - 27mg

Sodium - 31mg

Carbohydrate - 4.7g

Dietary Fiber - 0.7g

Sugars - 0.8g

Protein - 3.2g

Calcium - 68mg

Phosphorous - 120mg

Potassium - 100mg

Blackberry Cream Cheese Pie

Preparation Time: 5 minutes

Cooking Time: 45 minutes

Servings: 8

Ingredients:

⅓ cup of unsalted butter

4 cups of blackberries

1 teaspoon of stevia

1 cup of flour

½ teaspoon of baking powder

¾ cup of cream cheese

Directions:

- ➢ Switch your gas oven to 375°F to preheat.
- ➢ Layer a 2-quart baking dish with melted butter.
- ➢ Mix the blackberries with stevia in a small bowl.
- ➢ Beat the remaining ingredients in a mixer until they form a smooth batter.
- ➢ Evenly spread this pie batter in the prepared baking dish and top it with blackberries.
- ➢ Bake the blackberry pie for about 45 minutes in the preheated oven.
- ➢ Slice and serve once chilled.

Nutrition:

Calories - 239

Total Fat - 8.4g

Saturated Fat - 4.9g

Cholesterol - 20mg

Sodium - 63mg

Carbohydrate - 26.2g

Dietary Fiber - 4.5g

Sugars - 15.1g

Protein - 2.8g

Calcium - 67mg

Phosphorous - 105mg

Potassium - 170mg

Apple Cinnamon Pie

Preparation Time: 10 minutes

Cooking Time: 45 minutes

Servings: 12

Ingredients (apple filling):

9 cups of peeled, cored and sliced apples

1 tablespoon of stevia

⅓ cup of all-purpose flour

2 tablespoons of lemon juice

1 teaspoon of ground cinnamon

2 tablespoons of butter

Ingredients (pie dough):

2¼ cups of all-purpose flour

1 teaspoon of stevia

1½ sticks of unsalted butter

6 oz. of cream cheese

3 tablespoons of cold heavy whipping cream

Water (if needed)

Directions:

➢ Start by preheating your gas oven at 425°F.
➢ Mix the apple slices with cinnamon, 1 tablespoon of butter, lemon juice, flour and stevia in a bowl, and keep it aside covered.
➢ Whisk the flour with stevia, butter, cream cheese and cream in mixing bowl to form the dough.
➢ If the dough is too dry, slowly add some water to make a smooth dough ball.
➢ Cut the dough into two equal-size pieces and spread them into a 9-inch sheet.
➢ Place one of the sheets at the bottom of a 9-inch pie pan.
➢ Evenly spread the apples in this pie shell and add a tablespoon of butter over it.
➢ Cover the apple filling with the second sheet of the dough and pinch down the edges.
➢ Make 1-inch deep cuts on top of the pie and bake for about 50 minutes until golden.
➢ Slice and serve.

Nutrition:

Calories – 303 Total Fat - 8.8g Saturated Fat - 5.3g Cholesterol - 26mg Sodium - 30mg

Carbohydrate - 21.7g Dietary Fiber - 4.8g Sugars - 19.6g Protein - 4.2g Calcium - 21mg

Phosphorous - 381mg Potassium - 229mg

Cherry Pie Dessert

Cooking Time: 40 minutes

Servings: 8

Ingredients:

½ cup of unsalted butter

2 eggs

1 cup of granulated Swerve

1 cup of sour cream

1 teaspoon of vanilla

2 cups of all-purpose flour

1 teaspoon of baking powder

1 teaspoon of baking soda

20 oz. of cherry pie filling

Directions:

➢ First, begin by setting your gas oven at 350°F.
➢ Soften the butter first, then beat it with the cream eggs, swerve, vanilla and sour cream in a mixer.
➢ Separately mix the flour with the baking soda and baking powder.
➢ Add this mixture to the egg mixture, then mix well until smooth.
➢ Spread the batter evenly in a 9x13 inch baking pan.
➢ Bake the pie for 40 minutes in the oven until golden from the surface.
➢ Slice and serve with cherry pie filling on top.

Nutrition:

Calories - 470

Total Fat - 19g

Saturated Fat - 11.4g

Cholesterol - 84mg

Sodium - 285mg

Carbohydrate - 43.2g

Dietary Fiber - 1.3g

Sugars - 14.9g

Protein - 5.9g

Calcium - 82mg

Phosphorous - 249mg

Potassium - 232mg

CHAPTER 15:

28 Days Meal Plan

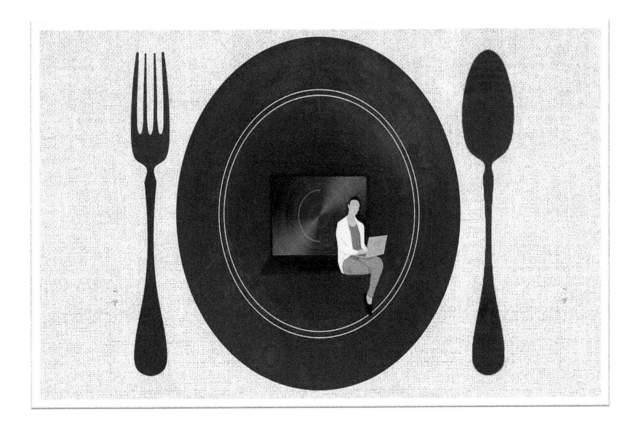

DAY	BREAKFAST	LUNCH	DINNER	DESSERT
1	Breakfast Tacos	Beef Brisket	Jambalaya	Strawberry Pizza
2	Citrus Pineapple Smoothie	Fish Taco	Rosemary Chicken	Quick Quiche
3	Summer Veggie Omelet	Pork Souvlaki	Cauliflower and Asparagus Tortilla	Grilled Peach Sundaes
4	Protein Berry Smoothie	Bagel with Salmon and Egg	Pork Loins with Leeks	Blueberry Cream Cones
5	Spiced French Toast	Fish with Mushrooms	Baked Eggplant Tray	Apple Cinnamon Pie
6	Apple Pumpkin Muffins	Apricot and Lamb Tagine	Broiled Shrimp	Cherry Dessert
7	Mango Lassi Smoothie	Carrot & Ginger Noodles	Spiced Lamb Burgers	Maple Crisp Bars
8	Mexican Style Burritos	Lemon & Herb Chicken Wraps	Grilled Squash	Pumpkin Cinnamon Roll
9	Vegetable Omelet	Shrimp in Garlic Sauce	Thai Tofu Broth	Cherry Coffee Cake
10	American Blueberry Pancakes	Ginger & Bean Sprout Steak Stir-Fry	Smokey Turkey Chili	Belgian Waffle with Fruits
11	Raspberry Smoothie	Chinese Beef Wraps	Mediterranean Veggie Pita Sandwich	Spicy Broccoli with Macaroni
12	Raspberry Overnight Porridge	Beef Chili	Avocado-Orange Grilled Chicken	Chocolate Trifle
13	Citrus Pineapple Shake	Baked Trout	Marinated Shrimp Pasta Salad	Maple Crisp Bars
14	Breakfast Maple Sausage	Chicken Meatloaf with Veggies	Eggplant Seafood Casserole	Cherry Dessert

15	Mango Lassi Smoothie	Fish with Mushrooms	Spiced Lamb Burgers	Quick Quiche
16	Vegetable Omelet	Ginger & Bean Sprout Steak Stir-Fry	Pork Loins with Leeks	Chocolate Trifle
17	Protein Berry Smoothie	Chinese Beef Wraps	Broiled Shrimp	Strawberry Pizza
18	American Blueberry Pancakes	Carrot & Ginger Noodles	Avocado-Orange Grilled Chicken	Belgian Waffle with Fruits
19	Raspberry Overnight Porridge	Apricot and Lamb Tagine	Thai Tofu Broth	Apple Cinnamon Pie
20	Citrus Pineapple Smoothie	Baked Trout	Baked Eggplant Tray	Spicy Broccoli with Macaroni
21	Apple Pumpkin Muffins	Beef Chili	Eggplant Seafood Casserole	Pumpkin Cinnamon Roll
22	Breakfast Maple Sausage	Bagel with Salmon and Egg	Rosemary Chicken	Cherry Coffee Cake
23	Breakfast Tacos	Chicken Meatloaf with Veggies	Grilled Squash	Blueberry Cream Cones
24	Mexican Style Burritos	Fish Taco	Jambalaya	Strawberry Pizza
25	Citrus Pineapple Shake	Shrimp in Garlic Sauce	Cauliflower and Asparagus Tortilla	Blueberry Cream Cones
26	Spiced French Toast	Pork Souvlaki	Marinated Shrimp Pasta Salad	Grilled Peach Sundaes
27	Raspberry Smoothie	Lemon & Herb Chicken Wraps	Broiled Shrimp	Belgian Waffle with Fruits
28	Summer Veggie Omelet	Beef Brisket	Mediterranean Veggie Pita Sandwich	Chocolate Trifle

Conclusion

Renal diet may seem restricting for many, but in reality, there are plenty of low-sodium, low-phosphorus and low-potassium options to try out, and we have proven it with this recipe book.

Keep in mind that we have included the approximate levels of all these minerals in every recipe. It is now your responsibility to calculate the total amounts you consume each day with all your daily meals.

Generally, most experts recommend a daily intake of up to 2700 mg of potassium and same amount of phosphorus for patients at the first two stages of renal disease. Those at a more advanced stage should aim to consume up to 2000mg each of these two minerals per day to avoid dialysis. Since most of the recipes featured in this e-book contain about 250 mg each of potassium and phosphorus, you can eat your breakfast, lunch and dinner without worrying about crossing your daily limits.

Don't forget to undergo regular medical check-ups to monitor your progress.

Good luck!

CPSIA information can be obtained
at www.ICGtesting.com
Printed in the USA
LVHW060753060121
675397LV00012B/893